W9-BFH-465

Guidelines for safe recreational water environments

VOLUME 2: SWIMMING POOLS AND SIMILAR ENVIRONMENTS

WORLD HEALTH ORGANIZATION

2006

WHO Library Cataloguing-in-Publication Data

World Health Organization.
   Guidelines for safe recreational water environments. Volume 2, Swimming pools
   and similar environments.

   1.Swimming pools — standards 2.Water quality — analysis 3.Drowning — prevention and
   control 4.Wounds and injuries — prevention and control 5.Risk management 6.Reference
   values 7.Guidelines I.Title II.Title: Swimming pools and similar environments.

   ISBN 92 4 154680 8   (NLM classification: WA 820)

© **World Health Organization 2006**

All rights reserved. Publications of the World Health Organization can be obtained from WHO Press, World Health
Organization, 20 Avenue Appia, 1211 Geneva 27, Switzerland (tel.: +41 22 791 2476; fax: + 41 22 791 4857; email:
bookorders@who.int). Requests for permission to reproduce or translate WHO publications – whether for sale or
for noncommercial distribution – should be addressed to WHO Press, at the above address (fax: +41 22 791 4806;
email: permissions@who.int).

The designations employed and the presentation of the material in this publication do not imply the expression of
any opinion whatsoever on the part of the World Health Organization concerning the legal status of any country,
territory, city or area or of its authorities, or concerning the delimitation of its frontiers or boundaries. Dotted lines
on maps represent approximate border lines for which there may not yet be full agreement.

The mention of specific companies or of certain manufacturers' products does not imply that they are endorsed or
recommended by the World Health Organization in preference to others of a similar nature that are not mentioned.
Errors and omissions excepted, the names of proprietary products are distinguished by initial capital letters.

All reasonable precautions have been taken by the World Health Organization to verify the information contained in
this publication. However, the published material is being distributed without warranty of any kind, either express
or implied. The responsibility for the interpretation and use of the material lies with the reader. In no event shall
the World Health Organization be liable for damages arising from its use.

Design by minimum graphics
Typeset by Strategic communications SA, Geneva
Printed in France

Contents

CHAPTER 4. CHEMICAL HAZARDS   **60**

CHAPTER 5. MANAGING WATER AND AIR QUALITY 80

CHAPTER 6. GUIDELINE IMPLEMENTATION 100

APPENDIX 1. LIFEGUARDS 114

List of acronyms and abbreviations

AFR	accidental faecal release
AIDS	acquired immunodeficiency syndrome
BCDMH	bromochlorodimethylhydantoin
BDCM	bromodichloromethane
cfu	colony-forming unit
CPR	cardiopulmonary resuscitation
CPSC	Consumer Product Safety Commission (USA)
DBAA	dibromoacetic acid
DBAN	dibromoacetonitrile
DBCM	dibromochloromethane
DBP	disinfection by-products
DCAA	dichloroacetic acid
DCAN	dichloroacetonitrile
DMH	dimethylhydantoin
FAO	Food and Agriculture Organization of the United Nations
GAE	granulomatous amoebic encephalitis
HAA	haloacetic acid
HIV	human immunodeficiency virus
HPC	heterotrophic plate count
HUS	haemolytic uraemic syndrome
HVAC	heating, ventilation and air conditioning
ID_{50}	infectious dose for 50% of the population
ILSF	International Life Saving Federation
ISO	International Organization for Standardization
JECFA	Joint FAO/WHO Expert Committee on Food Additives and Contaminants
LOAEL	lowest-observed-adverse-effect level
MBAA	monobromoacetic acid
MCAA	monochloroacetic acid
NOAEL	no-observed-adverse-effect level
NOEL	no-observed-effect level
NTU	nephelometric turbidity unit
ORP	oxidation–reduction potential
PAM	primary amoebic meningoencephalitis
pfu	plaque-forming unit
QMRA	quantitative microbiological risk assessment
TCAA	trichloroacetic acid

TCAN	trichloroacetonitrile
TDI	tolerable daily intake
TDS	total dissolved solids
THM	trihalomethane
TOC	total organic carbon
UFF	ultrafine filter
UV	ultraviolet
WHO	World Health Organization

Preface

The World Health Organization (WHO) has been concerned with health aspects of the management of water resources for many years and publishes various documents concerning the safety of the water environment and its importance for health. These include a number of normative "guidelines" documents, such as the *Guidelines for Drinking-water Quality* and the *Guidelines for the Safe Use of Wastewater, Excreta and Greywater*. Documents of this type are intended to provide a basis for standard setting. They represent a consensus view among experts on the risk to health represented by various media and activities and on the effectiveness of control measures in protecting health. They are based on critical review of the available evidence. Wherever possible and appropriate, such guideline documents also describe the principal characteristics of the monitoring and assessment of the safety of the medium under consideration as well as the principal factors affecting decisions to be made in developing strategies for the control of the health hazards concerned.

The *Guidelines for Safe Recreational Water Environments* are published in two volumes:

- *Volume 1: Coastal and Fresh Waters* provides an authoritative referenced review and assessment of the various health hazards encountered during recreational use of coastal and freshwater environments. It includes the derivation of guideline values or conditions and explains the basis for the decision to derive or not to derive them. It addresses a wide range of types of hazard, including hazards leading to drowning and injury, water quality, exposure to heat, cold and sunlight, and dangerous aquatic organisms; and provides background information on the different types of recreational water activity (swimming, surfing, etc.) to enable informed readers to interpret the Guidelines in light of local and regional circumstances. With regard to water quality, separate chapters address microbial hazards, freshwater algae, marine algae and chemical aspects. The volume describes prevention and management options for responding to identified hazards.

- *Volume 2: Swimming Pools and Similar Recreational Water Environments* provides an authoritative referenced review and assessment of the health hazards associated with recreational waters of this type; their monitoring and assessment; and activities available for their control through education of users, good design and construction, and good operation and management. The Guidelines include both specific guideline values and good practices. They address a wide range of types of hazard, including hazards leading to drowning and injury, water quality, contamination of associated facilities and air quality.

The preparation of this volume of *Guidelines for Safe Recreational Water Environments* has covered a period of over a decade and has involved the participation of numerous institutions and more than 60 experts from 20 countries worldwide. The work of the individuals concerned (see Acknowledgements) was central to the completion of the work and is much appreciated.

Acknowledgements

The assistance of the following persons in the development of the *Guidelines for Safe Recreational Water Environments, Volume 2: Swimming Pools and Similar Environments*, either in contribution of text or through provision of comments and constructive criticism, is appreciated:

Houssain Abouzaid, WHO Regional Office for the Eastern Mediterranean, Cairo, Egypt

Gabrielle Aggazzotti, University of Modena, Modena, Italy

Jamie Bartram, WHO, Geneva, Switzerland

Joost Bierens, VU University Medical Centre, Amsterdam, The Netherlands

Lucia Bonadonna, Istituto Superiore di Sanità, Rome, Italy

Christine Branche, National Center for Injury Prevention and Control, US Centers for Disease Control and Prevention, Atlanta, GA, USA

B. Chris Brewster, International Life Saving Federation, San Diego, CA, USA

Teresa Brooks, Health Canada, Ottawa, Canada

Marilyn L. Browne, Bureau of Environmental and Occupational Epidemiology, New York State Department of Health, Troy, NY, USA

Rudy Calders, Provinciaal Instituut voor Hygienne, Antwerp, Belgium

Richard Carr, WHO, Geneva, Switzerland

Rodney Cartwright, Microdiagnostics, Guildford, UK

Maurizio Cavalieri, Azienda Comunale Energia e Ambiente (ACEA), Rome, Italy

Paul C. Chrostowski, CPF Associates, Takoma Park, MD, USA

Joseph Cotruvo, NSF International, Washington, DC, USA

Carvin DiGiovanni, National Spa and Pool Institute, Alexandria, VA, USA

Alfred P. Dufour, National Exposure Research Laboratory, US Environmental Protection Agency, Cincinnati, OH, USA

Takuro Endo, National Institute of Infectious Diseases, Tokyo, Japan

Lothar Erdinger, Institute for Hygiene, University of Heidelberg, Germany

G. Fantuzzi, University of Modena, Modena, Italy

Norman Farmer, International Life Saving Federation, Melbourne, Australia

John Fawell, Independent Consultant, Flackwell Heath, UK

Lorna Fewtrell, Centre for Research into Environment and Health (CREH), University of Wales, Aberystwyth, UK

Maria Jose Figueras, University Rovira and Virgili, Tarragona-Reus, Spain

Willie Grabow, University of Pretoria, Pretoria, South Africa

Brian Guthrie, Pool Water Treatment Advisory Group, Norfolk, UK

Rudy Hartskeerl, Royal Tropical Institute (KIT), Amsterdam, The Netherlands

Christiane Höller, Bavarian Health and Food Safety Authority, Oberschleißheim, Germany

Paul Hunter, University of East Anglia, Norwich, UK

Owen Hydes, Independent Consultant, Mannings Heath, UK

Pranav Joshi, National Environment Agency, Singapore

Mihaly Kadar, National Institute of Hygiene, Budapest, Hungary

Simon Kilvington, Department of Microbiology and Immunology, University of Leicester, Leicester, UK

Tom Kuechler, Occidental Chemical Corporation, Sanget, IL, USA

Athena Mavridou, Technological Educational Institution of Athens, Athens, Greece

Charles Mbogo, Kenya Medical Research Institute, Kilifi, Kenya

Douglas B. McGregor (formerly of International Programme on Chemical Safety), Independent Consultant, Lyon, France

Art Mittelstaedt, Recreational Safety Institute, New York, NY, USA

Eric Mood, School of Medicine, Yale University, New Haven, CT, USA

Phil Penny, Independent Consultant, Taunton, UK

Kathy Pond, Robens Centre for Public and Environmental Health, University of Surrey, Guildford, Surrey, UK (formerly of WHO European Centre for Environment and Health, Rome, Italy)

Terry Price, TP Pool Water Treatment Services Ltd., Broxbourne, UK

M. Rayer, NSF International, Ann Arbor, MI, USA

Gareth Rees, Askham Bryan College, York, UK

R.G. Rice, RICE International Consulting Enterprises, Ashton, MD, USA

Ralph Riley, Institute of Sport and Recreation Management, Loughborough, UK

Will Robertson, Health Canada, Ottawa, Canada

Henry Salas, Pan American Center for Sanitary Engineering and Environmental Science, Lima, Peru

Ian Scott, WHO, Geneva, Switzerland

Geoff Shute, Tintometer Ltd., Salisbury, UK

Jeff Sloan, Chlorine Chemistry Council, Arlington, VA, USA

Jeff Soller, National Center for Environmental Assessment, US Environmental Protection Agency, Washington, DC, USA

Thor-Axel Stenström, Swedish Institute for Infectious Disease Control, Stockholm, Sweden

Paul Stevenson, Stevenson & Associates Pty Ltd., Sydney, Australia

Ernst Stottmeister, Federal Environment Agency (UBA), Bad Elster, Germany

Susanne Surman-Lee, Health Protection Agency, London, UK

Laura Tew, Arch Chemicals, Charleston, TN, USA

Carolyn Vickers, WHO, Geneva, Switzerland

Albrecht Wiedenmann, Baden-Württemberg State Health Office, Stuttgart, Germany

Adam Wooler, Royal National Lifeboat Institution, Saltash, Cornwell, UK (formerly of the Surf Life-Saving Association of Great Britain, Plymouth, Devon, UK)

Peter Wyn-Jones, University of Wales, Aberystwyth, UK

The preparation of these Guidelines would not have been possible without the generous support of the following, which is gratefully acknowledged: the European Commission; the States of Jersey, United Kingdom; the Department of the Environment, Transport and the Regions of the United Kingdom; the Ministry of Health of Germany; the Ministry of Environment of Germany; the Ministry of Health of Italy;

the Swedish International Development Cooperation Agency; and the United States Environmental Protection Agency.

Thanks are also due to Lorna Fewtrell for editing the complete text of the Guidelines and overseeing the review process and finalization of the Guidelines, Marla Sheffer for editing the initial draft and Grazia Motturi, Penny Ward, Windy Gancayo-Prohom and Evelyn Kortum-Margot for providing secretarial and administrative support.

Executive summary

This volume of the *Guidelines for Safe Recreational Water Environments* describes the present state of knowledge regarding the impact of the recreational use of swimming pools and similar environments upon the health of users – specifically drowning and injury, microbial contamination and exposure to chemicals. Control and monitoring of the hazards associated with these environments are discussed.

The primary aim of the Guidelines is the protection of public health. The purpose of the Guidelines is to ensure that swimming pools and similar recreational water facilities are operated as safely as possible in order that the largest possible population gets the maximum possible benefit and not to deter the use of these recreational water environments.

The Guidelines are intended to be used as the basis for the development of approaches to controlling the hazards that may be encountered in recreational water environments. The information provided is generally applicable to pools supplied with fresh, marine or thermal water, whether they are indoors or outdoors; public, semi-public or domestic; supervised or unsupervised. Information also relates to public, semi-public and domestic hot tubs (which, for the purposes of these Guidelines, is the term used to encompass a variety of facilities that are designed for sitting in, contain treated water usually above 32 °C, are often aerated and are not drained, cleaned and refilled for each user) and natural spas (facilities using thermal and/or mineral water). Although bathing houses, such as hammams, are not specifically covered, the principles outlined in the Guidelines should also be generally applicable to these environments. The preferred approaches adopted by national or local authorities towards implementation of guideline values and conditions may vary between these types of environment.

A guideline can be:

- a level of management;
- a concentration of a constituent that does not represent a significant risk to the health of members of significant user groups;
- a condition under which exposures with a significant risk are unlikely to occur; or
- a combination of the last two.

When a guideline is exceeded, this should be a signal to investigate the cause of the failure and identify the likelihood of future failure, to liaise with the authority responsible for public health to determine whether immediate action should be taken to reduce exposure to the hazard, and to determine whether measures should be put in place to prevent or reduce exposure under similar conditions in the future.

Drowning and injury prevention

Drowning, which is defined in these Guidelines as death arising from impairment of respiratory function as a result of immersion in liquid, is a major cause of death worldwide. Near-drowning is also a serious problem, as it may have lifelong effects. The recovery rate from near-drowning may be lower among young children than among teenagers and adults. Studies show that the prognosis for survival depends more on the effectiveness of the initial rescue and resuscitation than on the quality of subsequent hospital care. Most studies of accidental drowning have focused on children, and in some countries drowning is the leading cause of injury deaths among younger age groups. It has been suggested that in terms of swimming pools and similar environments most drownings occur in domestic pools and hot tubs, many while the child's supervisor assumed the child was safely indoors.

In swimming pools and similar environments, alcohol consumption is one of the most frequently reported contributory factors associated with drownings and near-drownings for adults, whereas lapses in parental supervision are most frequently cited for incidents involving children. Also of concern is the danger of drownings and near-drownings due to inlets and outlets where the suction is strong enough to cause entrapment of body parts or hair, causing the victim's head to be held under water.

Few preventive measures for drowning and near-drowning have been evaluated, although installation of isolation fencing around outdoor pools has been shown by some studies to decrease the number of pool immersion injuries by more than 50%. Pool fences around domestic pools should have a self-closing and self-latching gate and should isolate the pool. Barrier fencing should be at least 1.2 m high and have no hand- or footholds that could enable a young child to climb it. Fence slats should be no more than 10 cm apart. Above-ground pools should have steps or ladders leading to the pool that can be secured and locked to prevent access when the pool is not in use. For domestic or outdoor hot tubs, it is recommended that locked safety covers be used when the hot tub is not in use.

Preventive measures for hair and body entrapment in pools and similar environments include the use of grilles on drain gates that prevent hair entrapment, dual drains, an accessible and/or pressure-activated emergency shut-off for the pump and the wearing of bathing caps. Warnings displayed in the form of clear and simple signs as well as water safety instruction and adult supervision all may have value as preventive actions.

Of sports-related spinal cord injuries, the majority appear to be associated with diving. Injuries in diving incidents are almost exclusively located in the cervical vertebrae, resulting in quadriplegia (paralysis affecting all four limbs) or paraplegia (paralysis of both legs). Data suggest that diving into the upslope of a pool bottom or into the shallow portion of the pool is the most common cause of spinal injuries in pools. Alcohol consumption may contribute significantly to the frequency of injury. Education and raising awareness appear to offer the most potential for diving injury prevention.

Other injuries associated with the use of swimming pools and similar environments include brain and head injuries and arm, hand, leg and foot/toe injuries. Expert opinion suggests that the latter are common and generally go unreported. Causes include slippery decks, uncovered drains, reckless water entry, running on decks, tripping on swimming aids left on the poolside and stepping on glass (from broken bottles).

Maintenance of surfaces (including appropriate waste disposal), supervision of pool users, providing appropriate warnings, ensuring good underwater visibility and pool safety education are among the actions that can reduce these incidents.

High temperatures in hot tubs, for example, can cause drowsiness, which may lead to loss of consciousness or to heat stroke and death, and it is recommended that water temperatures in hot tubs be kept below 40 °C. Exposure to low temperatures in plunge pools, which are used in conjunction with saunas or steam baths, may result in slowed heart beat, hypothermia, impaired coordination, loss of control of breathing, muscle cramps and loss of consciousness. Temperature extremes should be avoided by users with medical problems, pregnant women and young children. Educational displays and warning signs, warnings from pool staff and regulations on time limits for use can reduce these adverse outcomes.

Microbial hazards

The risk of illness or infection associated with swimming pools and similar recreational water environments is primarily associated with faecal contamination of the water. This may be due to faeces released by the bathers or contaminated source water or, in the case of outdoor pools, may be the result of direct animal contamination (e.g. from birds and rodents). Many of the outbreaks related to pools and similar environments have occurred because disinfection was not applied or was inadequate. Non-faecal human shedding into the pool water or surrounding area is also a potential source of pathogenic organisms.

Swimming pool-related outbreaks of illness are relatively infrequent, but have been linked to viruses, bacteria, protozoa and fungi. Viral outbreaks are most often attributed to adenovirus, although hepatitis A, norovirus and echovirus have also been implicated in pool-related disease outbreaks. It should be borne in mind that the evidence linking viral outbreaks to a pool is generally circumstantial, and the causative viruses have rarely been isolated from the water.

Shigella and *Escherichia coli* O157 are two related bacteria that have been linked to outbreaks of illness associated with swimming in pools. Symptoms of *E. coli* O157 infection include bloody diarrhoea (haemorrhagic colitis) and haemolytic uraemic syndrome (HUS), as well as vomiting and fever in more severe cases. HUS, characterized by haemolytic anaemia and acute renal failure, occurs most frequently in infants, young children and elderly people. Symptoms associated with shigellosis include diarrhoea, fever and nausea.

The risk of illness in swimming pools associated with faecally-derived protozoa mainly involves two parasites: *Giardia* and *Cryptosporidium*. These two organisms have a cyst or oocyst form that is highly resistant to both environmental stress and disinfectants. They also both have high infectivity and are shed in high densities by infected individuals. Giardiasis is characterized by diarrhoea, cramps, foul-smelling stools, loss of appetite, fatigue and vomiting, whereas symptoms of cryptosporidiosis include diarrhoea, vomiting, fever and abdominal cramps.

The control of viruses and bacteria in swimming pool water is usually accomplished by appropriate treatment, including filtration and the proper application of chlorine or other disinfectants. Episodes of gross contamination of pool water due to an accidental faecal release, however, cannot all be effectively controlled by normal treatment and disinfectant levels. Where pools or spas are not disinfected, accidental faecal releases present an even greater problem. The only approach to maintaining public health protection under conditions of an accidental faecal release is to prohibit the use of the pool until the potential contaminants are inactivated.

Pool operators can help prevent faecal contamination of pools by encouraging pre-swim showering and toilet use and, where possible, confining young children to pools small enough to drain in the event of an accidental faecal release. It is recommended that people with gastroenteritis not use public or semi-public facilities while ill or for at least a week after their illness.

As well as pathogenic enteric organisms, a number of infectious non-enteric organisms may be transferred through pool water and the surrounding environment via human shedding. Infected users can directly contaminate pool waters and the surfaces of objects or materials at a facility with primary pathogens (notably viruses or fungi) in sufficient numbers to lead to skin and other infections in users who subsequently come in contact with the contaminated water or surfaces. Opportunistic pathogens (notably bacteria) can also be shed from users and be transmitted via both surfaces and contaminated water. In addition, certain free-living aquatic bacteria and amoebae can grow in pool, hot tub or natural spa waters, in pool or hot tub components or facilities (including heating, ventilation and air-conditioning systems) or on other wet surfaces within the facility to a point at which they may cause a variety of respiratory, dermal or central nervous system infections or diseases.

Most of the legionellosis, an often serious infection caused by *Legionella* species, associated with recreational water use has been associated with public and semi-public hot tubs and natural spas. Natural spas (especially thermal water) and hot tub water and the associated equipment create an ideal habitat (warm, nutrient-containing aerobic water) for the selection and proliferation of *Legionella*. *Pseudomonas aeruginosa* is also frequently present in hot tubs, as it is able to withstand high temperatures and disinfectants and to grow rapidly in waters supplied with nutrients from users. In hot tubs, the primary health effect associated with the presence of *P. aeruginosa* is folliculitis, an infection of the hair follicles that may result in a pustular rash.

It is less easy to control the growth of *Legionella* spp. and *P. aeruginosa* in hot tubs than in pools, as the design and operation of hot tubs can make it difficult to achieve adequate residual disinfection levels in these facilities. Thus, in public and semi-public facilities, frequent monitoring and adjustment of pH and disinfectant levels are essential, as are programmed 'rest periods' to allow disinfectant levels to 'recover'. In addition, facility operators should require users to shower before entering the water and control the number of users and the duration of their exposure. Thorough cleaning of the area surrounding the hot tub on a frequent basis (e.g. daily), complete draining and cleaning of the hot tub and pipework on at least a weekly basis, frequent backwashing and filter inspection and good ventilation are all recommended control measures.

Molluscipoxvirus (which causes molluscum contagiosum), papillomavirus (which causes benign cutaneous tumours – verrucae), *Epidermophyton floccosum* and various species of fungi in the genus *Trichophyton* (which cause superficial fungal infections of the hair, fingernails or skin) are spread by direct person-to-person contact or indirectly, through physical contact with contaminated surfaces. As the primary source of these viruses and fungi in swimming pools and similar environments is infected bathers, the most important means of controlling the spread of the infections is educating the public about the diseases, including the importance of limiting contact between infected and non-infected people and medical treatment. Thorough frequent cleaning and disinfection of surfaces in facilities that are prone to contamination can also reduce the spread of the diseases.

Chemical hazards

Chemicals found in swimming pool water can be derived from a number of sources, namely the source water, deliberate additions such as disinfectants and pool users themselves (these include sweat, urine, soap residues, cosmetics and suntan oil).

There are three main routes of exposure to chemicals in swimming pools and similar environments: direct ingestion of the water, inhalation of volatile or aerosolized solutes and dermal contact and absorption through the skin. The amount of water ingested by swimmers and bathers will depend upon a range of factors, including experience, age, skill and type of activity. Experimental evidence suggests that water intake varies according to age and sex, with adult women ingesting the least and male children ingesting the most. Swimmers inhale from the atmosphere just above the water's surface, and the volume of air inhaled is a function of the intensity of effort and time. Inhalation exposure will be largely associated with volatile substances that are lost from the water surface, but will also include some inhalation of aerosols, within a hot tub (for example) or where there is significant splashing. Dermal exposure depends upon the period of contact with the water, water temperature and the concentration of the chemical.

The principal management-derived chemicals are disinfectants, added to minimize the risk to pool users from microbial contaminants. Coagulants may be added as part of the water treatment process to enhance the removal of dissolved, colloidal or suspended material. Acids and alkalis may also be added to the water in order to maintain an appropriate pH for optimal water treatment and also the comfort of bathers.

The chemical disinfectants that are used most frequently include chlorine (as a gas, hypochlorite or, generally for outdoor pools, chlorinated isocyanurates), chlorine dioxide, bromochlorodimethylhydantoin (BCDMH), ozone and ultraviolet (UV) radiation (with ozone and UV usually being used in combination with a chlorine- or bromine-based disinfectant). Practice varies widely around the world, as do the levels of chemicals that are currently considered to be acceptable in order to achieve adequate disinfection while minimizing user discomfort. It is recommended that acceptable levels of free chlorine continue to be set at the local level, but in public and semi-public pools these should not exceed 3 mg/l and in public and semi-public hot tubs should not exceed 5 mg/l. It is recommended that total bromine does not exceed 4 mg/l in public and semi-public pools and 5 mg/l in hot tubs. Where chlorinated isocyanurates are used, levels of cyanuric acid in pool water should not exceed 100 mg/l. Where ozone is used, an air quality guideline of 0.12 mg/m^3 is recommended in order to protect bathers and staff working in the pool building.

A number of disinfectants can react with other chemicals in the water to give rise to unwanted by-products, known as disinfection by-products. Most is known about the by-products that result from the reaction of chlorine with humic and fulvic acids, but there is evidence from model studies with amino acids that other organic substances will also give rise to a similar range of by-products. Although there is potentially a large number of by-products, the substances produced in the greatest quantities are trihalomethanes, of which chloroform is generally present in the greatest concentrations, and the haloacetic acids, of which di- and trichloroacetic acid are generally present in the greatest concentrations. Both chlorine and bromine will react with ammonia in the water (resulting from the presence of urine) to form chloramines (monochloramine, dichloramine and nitrogen trichloride) and bromamines.

Trihalomethanes have been considered more than other chlorination by-products, reflecting the level of available information. Concentrations vary as a consequence of the concentration of precursor compounds, chlorine dose, temperature and pH. Trihalomethanes are volatile in nature and can be lost from the surface of the water, so they are also found in the air above the pool.

The guideline values in the WHO *Guidelines for Drinking-water Quality* can be used to screen for potential risks arising from swimming pools and similar environments, while making appropriate allowance for the much lower quantities of water ingested, shorter exposure periods and non-ingestion exposure. Although there are data to indicate that the concentrations of chlorination by-products in swimming pools and similar environments may exceed the concentrations proposed by WHO for drinking-water, the evidence indicates that for reasonably well managed pools, concentrations less than the drinking-water guideline values can be consistently achieved. The risks from exposure to chlorination by-products in reasonably well managed swimming pools would be considered to be small and must be set against the benefits of aerobic exercise and the risks of microbial disease in the absence of disinfection. Nevertheless, competitive swimmers and pool attendants can experience substantial exposure to volatile disinfection by-products via inhalation and dermal absorption. The chloramines and bromamines, particularly nitrogen trichloride and nitrogen tribromide, which are both volatile, can give rise to significant eye and respiratory irritation in swimmers and pool attendants. The provisional guideline value for chlorine species, expressed as nitrogen trichloride, in the atmosphere of swimming pools and similar environments is 0.5 mg/m^3.

Managing water and air quality

The primary water and air quality health challenges are, in typical order of public health priority, controlling clarity to minimize injury hazard, controlling water quality to prevent the transmission of infectious disease and controlling potential hazards from disinfection by-products. All of these challenges can be met through the combination of the following factors: treatment (to remove particulates, pollutants and microorganisms), including disinfection and filtration; pool hydraulics (to ensure effective distribution of disinfectant throughout the pool and removal of contaminated water); addition of fresh water at frequent intervals (to dilute substances that cannot be removed from the water by treatment); cleaning (to remove biofilms from surfaces, sediments from the pool floor and particulates adsorbed to filter materials); and adequate ventilation of indoor facilities.

Pre-swim showering will help to remove traces of sweat, urine, faecal matter, cosmetics, suntan oil and other potential water contaminants. Where pool users normally shower before swimming, pool water is cleaner, easier to disinfect with smaller amounts of chemicals and thus more pleasant to swim in. All users should also be encouraged to use the toilets before bathing to minimize urination in the pool and accidental faecal releases.

Disinfection is part of the treatment process whereby pathogenic microorganisms are inactivated by chemical (e.g. chlorination) or physical (e.g. UV radiation) means such that they represent no significant risk of infection. Circulating pool water is disinfected during the treatment process, and the entire water body is disinfected by the application of a residual disinfectant (chlorine- or bromine-based), which partially inactivates agents added to the pool by bathers. The choice of disinfectant depends upon a number of factors, including safety, compatibility with the source water, type, size and location of the pool, bathing load and the operation of the pool.

The concentration of disinfection by-products can be controlled to a significant extent by minimizing the introduction of precursors though source water selection, good bather hygienic practices (e.g. pre-swim showering), maximizing their removal by well managed pool water treatment and replacement of water by the addition of fresh supplies (i.e. dilution of chemicals that cannot be removed). It is inevitable, however, that some volatile disinfection by-products (such as chloroform and nitrogen trichloride) may be produced in the pool water and escape into the air. This hazard can be managed to some extent through good ventilation of indoor pool buildings.

Filtration is important in ensuring a safe pool. If filtration is poor, water clarity will decline and drowning risks increase. Disinfection will also be compromised, as particles associated with turbidity can surround microorganisms and shield them from the action of disinfectants. Particulate removal through coagulation and filtration is important for removing *Cryptosporidium* oocysts and *Giardia* cysts and some other protozoa that are resistant to chemical disinfection. For identifying bodies at the bottom of the pool, a universal turbidity value is not considered appropriate, as much depends on the characteristics of the specific pool. Individual standards should be developed, based on risk assessment at each pool, but it is recommended that, as a minimum, it should be possible to see a small child at the bottom of the pool from the lifeguard position while the water surface is in movement. In terms of effective disinfection, a useful, but not absolute, upper-limit guideline for turbidity is 0.5 nephelometric turbidity units.

Coagulation, filtration and disinfection will not remove all pollutants. Swimming pool design should enable the dilution of pool water with fresh water. Dilution limits the build-up of pollutants from bathers (e.g. constituents of sweat and urine), disinfection by-products and various other dissolved chemicals. Pool operators should replace pool water as a regular part of their water treatment regime. As a general rule, the addition of fresh water to disinfected pools should not be less than 30 litres per bather.

Good circulation and hydraulics in the pool ensure that the whole pool is adequately served by filtered, disinfected water. Treated water must get to all parts of the pool, and polluted water must be removed – especially from areas most used and most polluted by bathers. It is recommended that 75–80% be taken from the surface (where the pollution is greatest), with the remainder taken from the bottom of the pool.

Accidental faecal releases may occur relatively frequently, although it is likely that most go undetected. A pool operator faced with an accidental faecal release or vomit in the pool water must act immediately. If the faecal release is solid, it should be retrieved quickly and discarded appropriately. The scoop used to retrieve the faeces should be washed carefully and disinfected after use. If residual disinfectant levels are satisfactory, no further action is necessary. Where the stool is runny (diarrhoea) or if there is vomit, the situation is likely to be more hazardous. The safest course of action in small pools or hot tubs is to evacuate users, drain, clean and refill. Where draining is not possible, the pool should be cleared of people immediately; as much of the material as possible should be collected, removed and disposed of to waste; disinfectant levels should be maintained at the top of the recommended range or shock dosing used; using a coagulant (if appropriate), the water should be filtered for six turnover cycles; and the filter should be backwashed.

In indoor facilities, it is important to manage air quality as well as water quality in swimming pools and similar recreational water environments. This is important not only for staff and user health, but also for their comfort and to avoid negative impacts on the building fabric, and building code ventilation rates should be adhered to.

Parameters that are easy and inexpensive to measure and of immediate operational health relevance (such as turbidity, disinfectant residual and pH) should be monitored most frequently and in all pool types.

For a conventional public or semi-public swimming pool with good hydraulics and filtration, operating within its design bathing load, experience has shown that adequate routine disinfection should be achieved with a free chlorine level of 1 mg/l throughout the pool. Lower free chlorine concentrations (0.5 mg/l or less) will be adequate when chlorine is used in combination with ozone or UV disinfection. Higher concentrations (up to 2–3 mg/l) may be required for hot tubs, because of higher bathing loads and higher temperatures. Total bromine concentrations should not exceed 4 mg/l in public and semi-public pools and 5 mg/l in hot tubs.

In public and semi-public pools, residual disinfectant concentrations should be checked by sampling the pool before it opens and during the opening period (ideally during a period of high bathing load). It is suggested that the residual disinfectant concentration in domestic pools be determined before use. If the routine test results are outside the recommended ranges, the situation should be assessed and action taken.

The pH value of swimming pool water (and similar environments) must be controlled to ensure efficient disinfection and coagulation, to avoid damage to the pool fabric and to ensure user comfort. The pH should be maintained between 7.2 and 7.8 for chlorine disinfectants and between 7.2 and 8.0 for bromine-based and other non-chlorine processes.

There is limited risk of significant microbial contamination and illness in a well managed pool or similar environment with an adequate residual disinfectant concentration, a pH value maintained at an appropriate level, well operated filters and frequent monitoring of non-microbial parameters. Nevertheless, samples of pool water from public and semi-public pools should be monitored at appropriate intervals for microbial parameters, including heterotrophic plate count, thermotolerant coliforms or *E. coli*, *Pseudomonas aeruginosa* and *Legionella*. The frequency of monitoring and the guideline values vary according to microbial parameter and the type of pool.

Guideline implementation

Recreational water activities can bring health benefits to users, including exercise and relaxation. Effective management can control potential adverse health consequences that can be associated with the use of unsafe recreational water environments.

Different stakeholders play different roles in the management of the recreational water environment for safety. The typical areas of responsibility may be grouped into four major categories, although there may be overlap between these and stakeholders with responsibilities falling within more than one category:

- *Design and construction.* People responsible for commissioning pools and similar environments, along with designers and contractors, should be aware of the requirements to ensure safe and enjoyable use of facilities. Many decisions taken at the design and construction phase will have repercussions on the ease with which safe operation can be ensured once the pool is in use.
- *Operation and management.* Facility operators play a key role and are responsible for the good operation and management of the recreational water environment. This should include the preparation of and compliance with a pool safety plan, which consists of a description of the system, its monitoring and maintenance, normal operating procedures, procedures for specified incidents, a generic emergency plan and an emergency evacuation procedure.
- *Public education and information.* Facility operators, local authorities, public health bodies, pool-based clubs and sports bodies can play an important role in ensuring pool safety through public education and providing appropriate and targeted information to pool users.
- *Regulatory requirements (including compliance).* National legislation may include different sets of regulations that will apply to swimming pools and similar recreational environments. Regulation may control, for example, the design and construction of pools, their operation and management and control of substances hazardous to health. Within regulations it is likely that there will be a requirement for the use of certified material and, possibly, staff registered to certain bodies. Local regulatory oversight can support the work of pool management and provide greater public health protection and public confidence. Inspections by the regulatory officials to verify compliance with the regulations are an important component of this oversight.

Successful implementation of the Guidelines will also require development of suitable capacities and expertise and the elaboration of a coherent policy and legislative framework.

CHAPTER 1
Introduction

This volume of the *Guidelines for Safe Recreational Water Environments* describes the present state of knowledge regarding the possible detrimental impacts of the recreational use of swimming pools and similar recreational water environments upon the health of users, as well as the monitoring and control of the hazards associated with these environments.

1.1 General considerations

The hazards that are encountered in swimming pools and similar environments vary from site to site, as does exposure to the hazards. In general, most available information relates to health outcomes arising from exposure through swimming and ingestion of water. In the development of these Guidelines, all available information on the different uses of water and routes of exposure was taken into consideration.

This chapter covers the structure of this volume of the *Guidelines for Safe Recreational Water Environments* and introduces definitions of pool types, pool users and so on. The hazards from drowning and injury are probably the most obvious hazards relating to pools and similar environments, although there are also less visible hazards, including those posed by microbes and chemicals. These are covered in Chapters 2, 3 and 4, respectively. Most pools and similar environments apply treatment in managing water quality to ensure that the water is of an acceptable clarity and microbial and chemical quality. This can encompass filtration, pH control and disinfection with a range of disinfectants. Managing water and air quality to minimize health risks is covered in Chapter 5, while the roles of various stakeholders, regulatory measures and guideline implementation are dealt with in Chapter 6. This volume of the *Guidelines for Safe Recreational Water Environments* is structured as shown in Figure 1.1.

The primary aim of the *Guidelines for Safe Recreational Water Environments* is the protection of public health. The use of swimming pools and similar recreational water environments – and the resulting social interaction, relaxation and exercise – is associated with benefits to health and well-being. The purpose of the Guidelines is to ensure that the pools and similar environments are operated as safely as possible in order that the largest possible population gets the maximum possible benefit.

The Guidelines are intended to be used as the basis for the development of approaches to controlling the hazards that may be encountered in swimming pools and similar recreational water environments, as well as providing a framework for policy-making and local decision-taking. The Guidelines may also be used as reference material for industries and operators preparing to develop facilities containing swimming

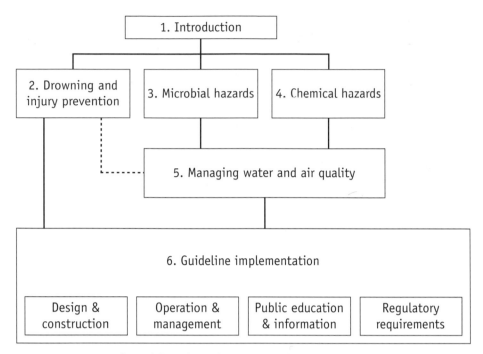

Figure 1.1. Structure of *Guidelines for Safe Recreational Water Environments, Vol. 2: Swimming Pools and Similar Environments*

pools and similar environments, as well as a checklist for understanding and assessing the potential health impacts of projects involving the development of such facilities.

The information provided in this volume of the Guidelines is intended to be generally applicable to public, semi-public (as encountered in clubs, hotels and schools, for example) and domestic (private) facilities (see Section 1.2). Although medical facilities (such as hydrotherapy pools) and bathing houses, such as hammams, are not specifically covered, the approaches outlined in these Guidelines should also be generally applicable to these environments. The preferred approaches adopted by national or local authorities towards implementation of guideline values and conditions may vary between these types of environment.

Because hazards may give rise to health effects after short- as well as long-term exposures, it is important that standards, monitoring and implementation enable preventive and remedial actions within real time frames. For this reason, emphasis in the Guidelines is placed upon identifying circumstances and procedures that are likely to lead to a continuously safe environment for recreation. This approach emphasizes monitoring of both conditions and practices and the use of threshold values for key indicators assessed through programmes of monitoring and assessment.

Concerned bodies – including national and local agencies, facility owners and operators, and nongovernmental organizations – have diverse management interventions. These range from proper facility planning to good operation and management practices, provision of appropriate levels of supervision (i.e. lifeguards), general educational activities to enhance awareness of health hazards and inform users on ways to avoid and respond to the hazards, and compliance with applicable regulatory requirements.

Where possible, numerical guideline values are presented as indicators of safety or good management (as described in Section 1.6). These guidelines use a risk–benefit approach. In the case of swimming pools and similar environments, development of such an approach concerns not only health risks, but also the health benefits and well-being derived from the recreational use of these environments. In developing strategies for the protection of public health, competent government authorities should take into account social, economic and environmental factors, including the general education of adults and children as well as the efforts and initiatives of nongovernmental organizations and industry operators in this area. This approach can often lead to the adoption of standards that are measurable and can be implemented and enforced. These would deal with, for example, water quality, safety of associated facilities and dissemination of information. A broad-based policy approach is required that will include legislation enabling positive and negative incentives to alter behaviour and monitor and improve situations. Such a broad base will require significant efforts in intersectoral coordination and cooperation at national and local levels, and successful implementation will require development of suitable capacities and expertise as well as the elaboration of a coherent policy and legislative framework.

1.2 Types of pools

Swimming pools may be supplied with fresh (surface or ground), marine or thermal water (i.e. from natural hot springs). They may be domestic (private), semi-public (e.g. hotel, school, health club, housing complex, cruise ship) or public (e.g. municipal), and they may be supervised or unsupervised. Swimming pools may be located indoors, outdoors (i.e. open air) or both; they may be heated or unheated. In terms of structure, the conventional pool is often referred to as the main, public or municipal pool. It is by tradition rectangular, with no extra water features (other than possible provision for diving), and it is used by people of all ages and abilities. There are also temporary or portable pools, which are often used in the domestic setting. In addition, there are many specialist pools for a particular user type – for example, paddling pools, learner or teaching pools, diving pools and pools with special features such as 'flumes' or water slides. Although termed swimming pools, they are often used for a variety of recreational activities, such as aqua-aerobics, scuba diving and so on (see Section 1.3).

Hot tubs, for the purposes of these Guidelines, is the term used to encompass a variety of facilities that are designed for sitting in (rather than swimming), contain water usually above 32 °C, are generally aerated, contain treated water and are not drained, cleaned or refilled for each user. They may be domestic, semi-public or public and located indoors or outdoors. A wide range of names is used for them, including spa pools, whirlpools, whirlpool spas, heated spas, bubble baths and Jacuzzi (a term that is used generically but is in fact a trade name).

Plunge pools are usually used in association with saunas, steam rooms or hot tubs and are designed to cool users by immersion in unheated water. They are usually only large enough for a single person, but can be larger. For the purposes of these Guidelines, they are considered to be the same as swimming pools.

Natural spa is the term used to refer to facilities containing thermal and/or mineral water, some of which may be perceived to have therapeutic value and because of certain water characteristics may receive minimal water quality treatment.

In addition, there are *physical therapy pools*, in which treatments for a variety of physical symptoms are performed by professionals on people with neurological, orthopaedic, cardiac or other diseases; these are termed 'hydrotherapy pools' and are defined as pools used for special medical or medicinal purposes. These are not specifically covered by the Guidelines, although many of the same principles that apply to swimming pools and hot tubs will also apply to hydrotherapy pools. There are also therapy pools containing small fish (*Garra ruffa*) that feed on the scaly skin lesions caused by psoriasis. These types of therapy pools are not covered by the Guidelines.

In many countries, there are public hygiene facilities to enable individuals and families to bathe. These are operated as drain and fill pools or baths and are not covered by these Guidelines.

Each type of pool has potentially different management problems, which must be anticipated and dealt with by pool managers. Of importance to the type of pool and its management is identification of how the pool will be used:

- the daily opening hours;
- the peak periods of use;
- the anticipated number and types of users; and
- special requirements, such as temperature, lanes and equipment.

The type, design and use of a pool may present certain hazards (e.g. pools may include sudden changes in depth, which may result in wading non-swimmers suddenly finding themselves out of their depth). Hot tubs, for example, may be subject to high bather loads relative to the volume of water. Where there are high water temperatures and rapid agitation of water, it may become difficult to maintain satisfactory pH, microbial quality and disinfectant concentrations.

In certain circumstances, in some natural spas utilizing thermal and mineral waters it may not be possible to treat the water in the usual way (i.e. by recycling or disinfection) because the agents believed to be of benefit, such as sulfides, would be eliminated or impaired. Also, chemical substances of geological origin in some types of deep thermal springs and artesian wells (such as humic substances and ammonium) may hamper the effect of disinfectants when these waters are used to fill pools without any pretreatment. These natural spas, therefore, require non-oxidative methods of water treatment (see Chapter 5). A very high rate of water exchange is necessary (even if not completely effective) if there is no other way of preventing microbial contamination, where complete drain-down between users is not possible.

Pools and hot tubs on ships are also a special case, as the source water may be either seawater or from the potable water supply for the ship. The hydraulic, circulation and treatment systems of the pool will necessitate a unique design in order to be able to deal with movement of the ship and the variable source water quality (outlined in more detail in WHO, 2005). They may also pose an increased risk of injury compared with land-based pools, especially when used in heavy seas.

1.3 Types of users
Users may include:

- the general public;
- children/babies;
- hotel guests;
- tourists;

- health club members;
- exercise class members (e.g. aqua-aerobics);
- competitive swimmers;
- non-swimmers;
- clients of outdoor camping parks;
- leisure bathers, including clients of theme parks; and
- specialist sporting users, including scuba divers, canoeists and water polo participants.

Certain groups of users may be more predisposed to hazards than others. For example:

- Children may spend long periods in recreational waters and are more likely than adults to intentionally or accidentally swallow water.
- The elderly and handicapped may have strength, agility and stamina limitations.
- Immunocompromised individuals may be at higher risk from microbial or chemical hazards.

1.4 Hazard and risk

Popularly, the terms hazard and risk are used interchangeably. Correctly, a *hazard* is a set of circumstances that could lead to harm – harm being injury, illness or loss of life. The *risk* of such an event is defined as the probability that it will occur as a result of exposure to a defined quantum of hazard. In simpler terms, hazard is the potential for harm, while risk is the chance that harm will actually occur. The *rate of incidence* or *attack rate* is the number of events expected to occur for this defined quantum of hazard. Strictly speaking, probabilities and rates obey different laws; however, if the probabilities are small and the events are independent, the two values will be approximately equal.

1.4.1 Types of hazard encountered

The most frequent hazards associated with the use of swimming pools and similar recreational water environments are:

- physical hazards (leading to, for example, drowning, near-drowning or injury);
- heat, cold and sunlight (see also WHO, 2003);
- water quality; and
- air quality.

Specific examples of the hazards and the associated adverse health outcomes are given in Table 1.1.

Drowning, near-drowning and spinal injury are severe health outcomes of great concern to public health. Human behaviour, especially alcohol consumption, is a prime factor that increases the likelihood of injuries. Other injuries, such as cuts and those arising from slip, trip and fall accidents, while less severe, cause distress and decrease the benefits to well-being arising from recreation. Preventive and remedial actions take diverse forms and include general education, posting of warnings where appropriate, the presence of lifeguards, use of non-slip surfaces, preventing the use of glass near the pool, preventing rough play or running poolside, the availability of health services such as first aid, the availability of communication with health and rescue services, and the cleaning of pools and associated facilities.

Table 1.1. Adverse health outcomes associated with hazards encountered in swimming pools and similar recreational water environments

Type of adverse health outcome	Examples of associated hazards (with chapter references in parentheses)
Drowning	Swimmers under the influence of alcohol, poor swimming ability, no supervision, poor pool design and maintenance (2).
Impact injuries	Impact against hard surfaces (2). The impact may be driven by the participant (diving, accidents arising from the use of water slides, collision, treading on broken glass and jagged metal – especially in outdoor pool surroundings).
Physiological	Acute exposure to heat and ultraviolet (UV) radiation in sunlight (refer to Volume 1 of the Guidelines – WHO, 2003). Cumulative exposure to sun for outdoor pool users (refer to Volume 1 of the Guidelines – WHO, 2003). Heat exposure in hot tubs or natural spas (using thermal water) or cold exposure in plunge pools (2).
Infection	Ingestion of, inhalation of or contact with pathogenic bacteria, viruses, fungi and protozoa, which may be present in water and pool surroundings as a result of faecal contamination, carried by participants or animals using the water or naturally present (3).
Poisoning, toxicoses and other conditions that may arise from long-term chemical exposures	Contact with, inhalation of or ingestion of chemically contaminated water, ingestion of algal toxins and inhalation of chemically contaminated air (4).

Much attention has focused in recent years upon microbial hazards. In particular, the health risks associated with contamination by excreta and associated gastroenteric outcomes have been the topic of both scientific and general public interest. Adverse health outcomes associated with microbial hazards also include skin, eye and ear infections arising from pollution of water by excreta from source waters and from bathers as well as non-enteric organisms arising from bathers or those naturally present in the aquatic environment.

Hazards to human health exist even in unpolluted environments. For example, eye irritation and some additional eye infections probably occur as a result of reduction in the eye's natural defences through limited contact with water and do not relate to water quality or pollution *per se*.

1.4.2 Assessment of hazard and risk

Assessments of hazard and risk inform the development of policies for controlling and managing risks to health and well-being in water recreation. Both draw upon experience and the application of common sense, as well as the interpretation of data.

Figure 1.2 provides a schematic approach to comparing health hazards encountered during recreational water use. A severe health outcome such as permanent paralysis or

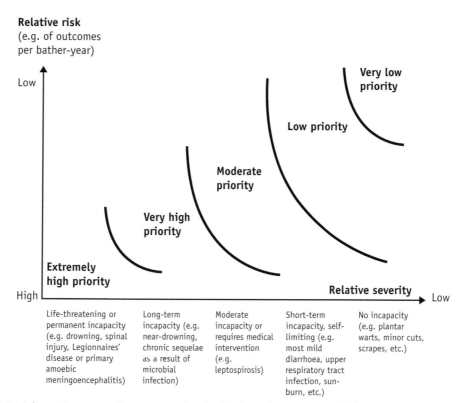

Relative risk
(e.g. of outcomes
per bather-year)

Low

**Very low
priority**

Low priority

**Moderate
priority**

**Very high
priority**

**Extremely
high priority**

High

Relative severity

Low

| Life-threatening or permanent incapacity (e.g. drowning, spinal injury, Legionnaires' disease or primary amoebic meningoencephalitis) | Long-term incapacity (e.g. near-drowning, chronic sequelae as a result of microbial infection) | Moderate incapacity or requires medical intervention (e.g. leptospirosis) | Short-term incapacity, self-limiting (e.g. most mild diarrhoea, upper respiratory tract infection, sun-burn, etc.) | No incapacity (e.g. plantar warts, minor cuts, scrapes, etc.) |

Figure 1.2. Schematic approach to comparing health hazards encountered during recreational water use

death, as a result of diving into shallow water, may affect only a small number of pool users annually but will warrant a high management priority. Minor skin irritations, encountered at the other end of the scale, may affect a higher number of users per year, but do not result in any significant incapacity, and thus require lower management priority. Figure 1.2 can be applied throughout the Guidelines. For each hazard discussed, the severity of the hazard can be related to the relative risk in the figure and can serve as a tool to initiate further research or investigation into the reduction of risk as well as to highlight or emphasize priority protective or remedial management measures.

Data on risk related to the use of swimming pools and similar recreational water environments take four main forms:

- national and regional statistics of illness and deaths;
- clinical surveillance of the incidence of illness and outbreaks;
- epidemiological studies and surveys; and
- accident and injury records held by facility owners/managers and local authorities.

Although 'incident records' held by local pools and authoritative bodies may be comprehensive, published statistics are seldom sufficiently detailed for risk assessment.

Systems for surveillance of public health operate in some countries. They serve the broad purpose of alerting either regulator or supplier to changes in incidence of disease and to the need for initiating immediate investigation of the causes and remedial action. Such investigation will involve epidemiology (the study of the occurrence and causes of disease in populations). Galbraith & Palmer (1990) give details of the use of epidemiology in surveillance. Epidemiology may also be used as a research tool to investigate hypotheses concerning the causes of illness.

There are other reasons why it is difficult to estimate risk directly, such as the following:

- In most active water sports, enjoyment arises from the use of skill to avoid and overcome perceived hazards. The degree of competence of participants and the use of properly designed equipment, accompanied by appropriate supervision and training, will considerably modify the risk.
- Risks of acquiring infectious disease will be influenced by innate and acquired immunity (for examples, see Gerba et al., 1996). The former comprises a wide range of biological and environmental factors (age, sex, nutrition, socioeconomic and geographic), as well as body defences (impregnability of the skin, lysozyme secretion in tears, mucus and sweat, the digestive tract and phagocytosis). Previous challenge by pathogens often results in transient or long-lasting immunity. Immunocompromised individuals will be at greater risk of acquiring infectious diseases (see Pond, 2005).
- Assessment of harm itself and the degree of harm suffered depends upon judgement at the time. Medical certification of injury and of physiological illness and infection, accompanied by clinical diagnosis, is the most reliable information. Information obtained by survey or questionnaire will contain a variable degree of uncertainty caused by the subjects' understanding of the questions, their memory of the events and any personal bias of the subject and interviewer. Survey information is only as good as the care that has gone into the design and conduct of the survey.
- The causes of harm must be ascertained as far as possible at the time. There are considerable difficulties in determining causes in the cases of low-level exposures to chemical and physical agents that have a cumulative or threshold effect and of infectious diseases caused by those pathogens that have more than one route of infection or have a long period of incubation. For example, gastroenteric infections at swimming pool facilities may result from person-to-person contact or faulty food hygiene in catering, as well as from ingesting pathogen-contaminated water.
- Where data are in the form of published regional or national statistics giving attack rates, the exact basis on which the data are collected and classified must be ascertained. For example, national statistics on deaths by drowning will usually include suicides, occupational accidents (e.g. lifeguards), natural disasters (e.g. flooding due to storm events) and misadventure in recreation.
- It cannot be assumed that risk is directly proportional to exposure or that risks from multiple exposures or a combination of different factors will combine additively.

1.4.3 Degree of water contact

For hazards where contact with water and ingestion of water are important, an understanding of the different degrees of contact associated with different pool types and uses is helpful. For example, the degree of water contact directly influences the amount of exposure to pathogens and toxic agents found in contaminated water and aerosols and therefore the likelihood of illness.

The degrees of water contact encountered in the many different types of swimming pools and similar recreational water environments may be classified as follows:

- *No contact* – for example, use of outdoor pools just for sunbathing and not swimming.
- *Meaningful direct contact* – involves a negligible risk of swallowing water, such as the use of a wading pool by adults.
- *Extensive direct contact* – with full body immersion and a significant risk of swallowing water, e.g. swimming, diving.

1.5 Measures to reduce risks

Reduction of most, if not all, of the health risks associated with the hazards described in Table 1.1 can be obtained by avoiding the circumstances giving rise to the hazard or by mitigating their effect. For example, glass left on the poolside may cause cuts to walkers with bare feet, which may be overcome by regular cleaning of the pool, excluding glass from the pool area, provision of litter bins and educational awareness campaigns. Accidents caused by misuse of water slides may be overcome by increased supervision by lifeguards and education of users regarding proper behaviour. Each type of recreational activity should be subject to a hazard assessment to determine what type of control measures will be most effective. Assessment should include modifying factors, such as local features, seasonal effects (for outdoor pools) and competence of the participants.

Controls for reducing risks in swimming pools and similar environments are discussed in Chapters 5 and 6. Different uses and types of pools involve different degrees of water contact and exposure to the various hazards. Measures for risk reduction will therefore be tailor-made to each pool type and to particular circumstances.

Management of swimming pools and similar recreational waters can be classified into four major categories (as described in Chapter 6):

- design and construction of facilities (including licensing and authorization, as appropriate);
- operation and management (including pool safety plan and lifeguard training);
- public education and information; and
- regulatory requirements (including licensing of equipment, chemicals, etc., available for use in swimming pools and similar environments).

1.6 Nature of the guidelines

A guideline can be a level of management, a concentration of a constituent that does not represent a significant risk to the health of members of significant user groups, a condition under which exposures associated with a significant risk are unlikely to occur, or a combination of the last two. In deriving guidelines including guideline values, account is taken of both the severity and frequency of associated health outcomes. Recreational water use areas conforming to the guidelines may, however, present a health risk to especially susceptible individuals or to certain user groups.

When a guideline is exceeded, this should be a signal to investigate the cause of the failure and identify the likelihood of future failure, to liaise with the authority responsible for public health to determine whether immediate action should be taken to reduce exposure to the hazard, and to determine whether measures should be put in place to prevent or reduce exposure under similar conditions in the future.

For most parameters, there is no clear cut-off value at which health effects are excluded, and the derivation of guidelines and their conversion to standards therefore include an element of valuation addressing the frequency and nature of associated health effects. This valuation process is one in which societal values play an important role. The conversion of guidelines into national policy, legislation and standards should therefore take account of environmental, social, cultural and economic factors.

Many of the hazards associated with swimming pools and similar recreational water environments may give rise to health effects after short-term exposures: accidents and exposures to microbial infective doses may occur in very short periods of time. Short-term deviations above guideline values or conditions are therefore of importance to health, and measures should be in place to ensure and demonstrate that recreational water environments are continuously safe during periods of actual or potential use.

This volume of the *Guidelines for Safe Recreational Water Environments* does not address:

- occupational exposures of individuals working in recreational water environments;
- waters afforded special significance for religious purposes and which are therefore subject to special cultural factors;
- therapeutic uses of water (hydrotherapy, balneotherapy or thalassotherapy);
- facilities, such as bathing houses, that are drained and refilled between users;
- risks associated with ancillary facilities that are not part of swimming pools and similar recreational water environments — thus, while poolside surfaces are addressed, toilet facilities in adjacent areas are not considered beyond assertion of the need for them in order to minimize soiling of the recreational environment;
- 'biopools', which are artificially created small 'lakes' (which can be either indoors or outdoors) that are sealed against groundwater and natural surface water influence and are becoming increasingly popular. In these pools the water is not disinfected but is circulated through 'regeneration' areas (reeds or soil filters);
- electrocution;
- hazards associated with UV radiation (from sunlight);
- aesthetic factors;
- beneficial effects, health claims, the efficacy of therapeutic use or the scale of health benefits arising from relaxation and exercise associated with recreational water use; or
- rescue, resuscitation or evacuation procedures from swimming pools and other recreational water facilities.

1.7 References

Galbraith S, Palmer S (1990) General epidemiology. In: Smith GR, Easmon CSF, eds. *Topley and Wilson's principles of bacteriology, virology and immunity. Vol. 3. Bacterial diseases*. London, Edward Arnold, pp. 11–29.

Gerba CP, Rose JB, Haas CN (1996) Sensitive populations: who is at the greatest risk? *International Journal of Food Microbiology*, 30(1–2): 113–123.

Pond K (2005) *Water recreation and disease: An expert review of the plausibility of associated infections, their acute effects, sequelae and mortality.* IWA on behalf of the World Health Organization, London, UK.

WHO (2003) *Guidelines for safe recreational water environments. Vol. 1. Coastal and fresh waters.* Geneva, World Health Organization, 219 pp.

WHO (2005) *Guide to ship sanitation.* Geneva, World Health Organization, in preparation.

CHAPTER 2

Drowning and injury prevention

A number of injuries may result from the use of swimming pools and similar recreational water environments. Prominent among them are:

- drowning and non-fatal or near-drowning;
- major impact injuries (spinal, brain and head injuries);
- slip, trip and fall injuries; and
- disembowelment.

This chapter addresses these adverse health outcomes, their causation and contributory factors, along with evidence concerning preventive measures.

2.1 Drowning

Drowning has been defined as death arising from impairment of respiratory function as a result of immersion in liquid, and this is the definition employed in these Guidelines. A wider definition of drowning includes outcomes ranging from no morbidity to morbidity to death (World Congress on Drowning, 2002). Drowning is a major cause of death, and it has been estimated that, in 2002, 382 million people drowned worldwide, with 97% of drownings occurring in low- and middle-income countries (Peden & McGee, 2003; WHO, 2004), although the majority of available data relate to developed countries. It is the third leading cause of death in children aged 1–5 and the leading cause of mortality due to injury, with the mortality rates in male children being almost twice as high as those in female children (Peden & McGee, 2003). Not all drownings are related to recreational water use, and the percentage that is attributable to swimming pools and similar environments is likely to vary from country to country.

Overall drowning statistics (i.e. not confined to swimming pools) for the USA, shown in Table 2.1, support the observation from numerous studies that children less than 5 years of age and young adults between the ages of 15 and 24 years have the highest drowning rates (e.g. Blum & Shield, 2000; Browne et al., 2003; Smith, 2005).

In the USA, an investigation into drownings in New York State residents (with a population of almost 18 million) between 1988 and 1994 found that there were on average 173 drownings a year (1210 over the seven-year period). A total of 883 non-bathtub drownings that took place in-state were included in the study. Of these, 156 (18%) took place in pools or hot tubs (Browne et al., 2003), with domestic pools predominating (123 cases). Almost 60% of drownings in children aged 0–4 years, however, occurred in swimming pools or hot tubs. Analysis of figures from the whole

Table 2.1. Drowning statistics for the USA (per 100 000)[a]

Ages (years)	1997		1996		1995	
	Deaths	Rates	Deaths	Rates	Deaths	Rates
0–4	516	2.69	533	2.76	596	3.05
5–9	234	1.19	223	1.15	222	1.16
10–14	215	1.13	225	1.19	242	1.29
15–19	349	1.83	388	2.08	442	2.43
20–24	316	1.80	327	1.86	348	1.93
25–29	298	1.58	291	1.53	292	1.54

[a] Adapted from National Center for Health Statistics, 1998

of the USA for 2001 reveals similar results, with 18% of fatal drownings occurring in swimming pools (CDC, 2004). In the State of Arizona, USA, 85% of emergency calls relating to drownings and near-drownings in children aged four or less were associated with swimming pools (CDC, 1990). In the United Kingdom, children are more likely to drown in natural water bodies (sea, lakes, etc.) than in swimming pools, although pools still account for a substantial proportion of drowning, with 19% of drowning deaths in children aged 0–14 years being attributable to pools in 1988–1989, and 11% in 1998–1999 (Sibert et al., 2002). These authors note, however, that at least 14 British children drowned while abroad, with most of these drownings occurring in hotel or apartment pools.

During a period of over 20 years (since 1980), the USA Consumer Product Safety Commission (CPSC) has received reports of more than 700 deaths in hot tubs. Approximately one third of these were drownings of children under five years of age (CPSC, undated).

Death by drowning is not the sole outcome of distress in the water. Near-drowning is also a serious problem. One study (Wintemute et al., 1987) found that for every 10 children who die by drowning, 140 are treated in emergency rooms and 36 are admitted to hospitals for further treatment (see also Spyker, 1985; Liller et al., 1993), although some never recover. In the Netherlands, it has been reported that on average there are about 300 drowning fatalities a year and an additional 450 cases who survive the drowning incident; of these, 390 are admitted to hospital for further treatment (Bierens, 1996). Browne et al. (2003) reported that there are on average 173 drownings among New York State residents every year, and it is estimated that there are 177 non-fatal hospitalizations. Analysis of data from the USA for 2001–2002 led to the estimation that about 4174 people on average each year are treated in hospital emergency departments for non-fatal drowning injuries in recreational water settings, over 65% of these cases occurred in swimming pools and over 52% were in children under the age of 5 (CDC, 2004).

The recovery rate from near-drowning may be lower among young children than among teenagers and adults. Some survivors suffer subsequent anoxic encephalopathy (Pearn et al., 1976; Pearn & Nixon, 1977) leading to long-term neurological deficits (Quan et al., 1989). Studies show that the prognosis depends more on the effectiveness of the initial rescue and resuscitation than on the quality of subsequent hospital care (Cummings & Quan, 1999).

2.1.1 Contributory factors

Males are more likely to drown than females (Browne et al., 2003; Peden & McGee, 2003). This is generally attributed to higher exposure to the aquatic environment and a higher consumption of alcohol (leading to decreased ability to cope and impaired judgement) and their inclination towards higher risk-taking activity (Dietz & Baker, 1974; Mackie, 1978; Plueckhahn, 1979; Nichter & Everett, 1989; Quan et al., 1989; Howland et al., 1996).

Alcohol consumption is one of the most frequently reported contributory factors associated with adolescent and adult drownings in many countries (Howland & Hingson, 1988; Levin et al., 1993; Browne et al., 2003; Petridou, 2005). Although the proportion of alcohol-related drownings is often not presented according to body of water (and swimming pools and hot tubs are the site of relatively few adult and adolescent drownings), in one study a blood alcohol screen was positive for approximately 50% of drowning victims over 14 years of age (M. Browne, pers. comm.). Among children, lapses in parental supervision are the most frequently cited contributory factor (Quan et al., 1989), although alcohol consumption by the parent or guardian may also play a role in the lapse of supervision (Petridou, 2005).

Browne et al. (2003) examined the means of access of young children involved in domestic swimming pool drownings. The following were found to be the most common:

- open or unlocked gate or ineffective latch;
- no fence, no separate fence (completely enclosing the pool area) or fence in disrepair;
- access directly from the house; and
- ladder to above-ground pool left in accessible 'down' position.

In this study, 43 of 77 (56%) of the drownings in children aged 0–4 occurred in the child's family pool, 17 (22%) occurred in the domestic pool of a relative and 8 (10%) occurred in a neighbour's domestic pool (M. Browne, pers. comm.).

In Australia, a similar study found that more than half of the children studied drowned in unfenced or unsecured pools and hot tubs. Where children gained access to fenced pools, most did so through faulty or inadequate gates or through gates that were propped open (Blum & Shield, 2000). Access has also infrequently been as a result of climbing onto objects next to the pool fence (e.g. pool filters).

While a high proportion of persons drowning are non-swimmers or poor swimmers (Spyker, 1985), there are conflicting opinions as to the role of swimming skills in preventing drowning and near-drowning (Patetta & Biddinger, 1988; Asher et al., 1995; Brenner, 2005). Hyperventilation before breath-hold swimming and diving has been associated with a number of drownings among individuals, almost exclusively males, with excellent swimming skills. Although hyperventilation makes it possible for a person to extend his or her time under water, it may result in a loss of consciousness by lowering the carbon dioxide level in the blood and decreasing the partial oxygen pressure in the arterial blood on surfacing (Craig, 1976; Spyker, 1985).

Inlets and outlets where the suction is extremely strong can trap body parts or hair, causing the victim's head to be held under water. Most accidents involve people with shoulder-length or longer hair. Hair entrapment occurs when the water flow into the inlet takes the bather's hair into and around the outlet cover, and the hair is pulled into the drain as a result of the suction created. In the USA, during a six and a half year period, between 1990 and 1996, the CPSC received reports of 49 incidents of hair entrapment/entanglement in hot tubs, 13 of which resulted in drowning (CPSC, undated). This suction problem may also occur in the main pool drains of swimming pools, but to a much lesser extent than with hot tubs.

A number of drowning deaths have also occurred after the body or a limb has been held against a drain by the suction of the circulation pump. In the USA, CPSC reported 18 cases of body entrapment over a 20-year period. Ten of these resulted in disembowelment (see Section 2.5), and five other cases were fatal (CPSC, undated). Young children, typically between the ages of 8 and 16 years, are particularly likely to play with open drains, inserting hands or feet into the pipe and then becoming trapped with the resulting suction. Any open drain or flat grating that the body can cover completely, combined with a plumbing layout that allows a build-up of suction if the drain is blocked, presents this hazard.

High temperatures (above 40 °C) in spas or hot tubs, especially in combination with alcohol consumption, may cause drowsiness, which may lead to unconsciousness and, consequently, drowning (Press, 1991).

Further contributory factors in drowning and near-drowning include:

- those related to the bather, such as a pre-existing health condition (e.g. seizure disorder – Ryan & Dowling, 1993);
- those related to the staff, such as lack of proper training for emergency response; and
- those related to the pool facility, such as water depth, water clarity, pool configuration and pool size.

Water clarity is particularly critical to water safety. If it is not possible to see the bottom of the pool at its deepest point, pool users and lifeguards may not be able to identify people in distress. In addition, a person entering the pool may not be able to see someone under the water or may not be able to judge the pool bottom configuration. Natural and artificial reflected light from the water surface may also affect vision in a similar way to poor water clarity. Swimming pool designers need to consider this when locating windows and designing lighting systems.

2.1.2 *Preventive and management actions*

It has been estimated that over 80% of all drownings can be prevented, and prevention is the key management intervention (World Congress on Drowning, 2002; Mackie, 2005). Surprisingly, there is no clear evidence that drowning rates are greater in poor swimmers (Brenner, 2005), and the value of swimming lessons and water safety instruction as drowning preventive measures has not been demonstrated (Patetta & Biddinger, 1988; Mackie, 2005). There is a significant debate regarding the age at which swimming skills may be safely acquired. The need for adult supervision is not decreased when young children acquire increased skills, and the possibility that training decreases parental vigilance has not been assessed (Asher et al., 1995). Lapses in supervision may make this an insufficient preventive measure alone (Quan et al., 1989).

Children should be taught to stay away from water and pools when unsupervised, but for outdoor pools, care must also be taken to prevent unauthorized entry (especially by young children). For domestic pools, barriers such as fences or walls will prevent some drownings by preventing a child from entering a swimming pool area unsupervised or may delay their entry long enough for the carer to realize they are missing.

Installation of isolation fencing around outdoor pools, which separates the pool from the remaining yard and house, has been shown in some studies to decrease the number of drownings and near-drownings by more than 50% (Pearn & Nixon, 1977; Milliner et al., 1980; Present, 1987). In Australia, Blum & Shield (2000) found that in the childhood drowning that they studied, no child had gained unaided access to a pool fitted with a fully functional gate and fence that met the Australian standard. A systematic review of studies (Thompson & Rivara, 2000) examining the effectiveness of pool fencing indicated that pool fencing significantly reduced the risk of drowning, with isolation fencing (enclosing the pool only) being superior to perimeter fencing (enclosing the pool and the property). The results of the review are supported by Stevenson et al. (2003). This study, conducted in Australia, found that during a 12-year period 50 children under the age of five drowned in domestic swimming pools and 68% of the drownings occurred in pools that did not have isolation fencing. Pool fences around domestic pools should have a self-closing and self-latching gate and should isolate the pool. Barrier fencing should be at least 1.2 m high and have no hand- or footholds that could enable a young child to climb it. Fence slats should be no more than 10 cm apart to prevent a child squeezing through, thus ensuring that the safety barrier itself is not a hazard. Above-ground pools should have steps or ladders leading to the pool that can be secured and locked to prevent access when the pool is not in use. Care should also be taken to ensure that poolside equipment is not positioned such that it may be used to climb the fence and access the pool. For domestic or outdoor hot tubs, it is recommended that locked safety covers be used when the hot tub is not in use.

Pool alarms and pool covers have not been shown to be reliable preventive measures for very young children. In fact, pool covers may themselves contribute to drowning – if they are not strong enough to hold the child's weight, the child could slip under the cover and be trapped by it, or the child could drown in small puddles of water formed on their surface. In addition, covers may delay the discovery of a drowning victim.

To prevent entrapment, it is recommended that the velocity of water flowing from the pool through outlets should not exceed 0.5 m/s and there should be a minimum of two outlets to each suction line. Also, they should be sized and located such that they cannot be blocked by the body of a single bather. Grilles in outlets should have gaps of less than 8 mm. In addition, pools and hot tubs should not be used if any of the covers are missing, unsecured or damaged.

The availability of cardiopulmonary resuscitation (CPR) (including infant and child CPR) skills (Patetta & Biddinger, 1988; Orlowski, 1989; Liller et al., 1993; Kyriacou et al., 1994; Pepe & Bierens, 2005) has been reported to be important in determining the outcome of potential drownings.

The principal contributory factors and preventive actions (some of which have received scientific evaluation) concerned with drowning and near-drowning are summarized in Table 2.2.

2.2 Spinal injury

Data concerning the number of spinal injuries sustained as a result of pool use are not widely available. Stover & Fine (1987) estimated the total prevalence of spinal cord injury in the USA to be around 906 per million, with an annual rate of incidence of around 30 new spinal cord injuries per million persons at risk, and according to the Think First Foundation (2004), USA, 10% of all spinal cord injuries are related to

Table 2.2. Drowning and near-drowning: Principal contributory factors and preventive and management actions

Contributory factors

- Falling unexpectedly into water
- Easy unauthorized access to pools
- Not being able to swim
- Alcohol consumption
- Excessive 'horseplay' or overexuberant behaviour
- Swimming outside the depth of the user
- Breath-hold swimming and diving
- High drain outlet suction and poor drain and drain cover design
- High water temperatures

Preventive and management actions

- Isolation fences with self-closing and self-latching gates around outdoor pools
- Locked steps/ladders for above-ground pools
- Locked doors for indoor pools
- Locked safety covers for domestic and outdoor hot tubs
- Continuous parental/caregiver supervision of children
- Provision of properly trained and equipped lifeguards
- Teaching children to stay away from water when unsupervised
- Education/public awareness that drowning can happen quickly and quietly
- Restriction of alcohol provision or supervision where alcohol is likely to be consumed
- Suction outlets cannot be sealed by single person, and at least two suction outlets per pump
- Accessible emergency shut-off for pump
- Grilles/pipes on drain gates preclude hair entrapment
- Wearing bathing caps
- Maintaining water temperature in hot tubs below 40 °C
- Access to emergency services

diving into water. In Ontario, Canada, Tator & Edmonds (1986) report that between 1948 and 1983, diving accounted for 58.9% of all recreational-related spinal cord injury – 60 major spinal injuries each year.

Blanksby et al. (1997) tabulated data from a series of studies concerning diving accidents as the cause of acute spinal injury in various regions of the world. In one study (Steinbruck & Paeslack, 1980), 212 of 2587 spinal cord injuries were sports related, 139 of which were associated with water sports, the majority (62%) with diving. Diving-related injuries were found to be responsible for between 3.8% and 14% of traumatic spinal cord injuries in a comparison of French, Australian, English and American studies (Minaire et al., 1983), for 2.3% in a South African study and for 21% in a Polish study (Blanksby et al., 1997).

In diving incidents of all types, spinal injuries are almost exclusively located in the cervical vertebrae (Minaire et al., 1983; Blanksby et al., 1997). Statistics such as those cited above therefore underestimate the importance of these injuries, which typically cause quadriplegia (paralysis affecting all four limbs) or, less commonly, paraplegia (paralysis of both legs). In Australia, for example, diving incidents account for approximately 20% of all cases of quadriplegia (Hill, 1984). The financial cost of these injuries to society is high, because persons affected are frequently healthy young people, typically males under 25 years of age (DeVivo & Sekar, 1997).

2.2.1 Contributory factors

Data from the USA suggest that diving into the upslope of a pool bottom or shallow water is the most common cause of spinal injuries in pools. Diving or jumping from trees, balconies and other structures is particularly dangerous, as are special dives such as the swan or swallow dive, because the arms are not outstretched above the head but are to the side of the body (Steinbruck & Paeslack, 1980). Familiarity with the pool may not necessarily be protective; in one study from South Africa (Mennen, 1981), it was noted that the typical injurious dive is into a water body known to the individual.

Minimum depths for safe diving are greater than is frequently perceived, but the role played by water depth has been debated. Inexperienced or unskilled divers require greater depths for safe diving. The velocities reached from ordinary dives are such that the sight of the bottom, even in clear water, may provide an inadequate time for deceleration response (Yanai et al., 1996).

Most diving injuries occur in relatively shallow water (1.5 m or less) and few in very shallow water (i.e. less than 0.6 m), where the hazard may be more obvious (Gabrielsen, 1988; Branche et al., 1991). In a sample of 341 persons with spinal injuries resulting from swimming pool incidents, over half of the injuries occurred when the individuals dived into less than 1.2 m of water (DeVivo & Sekar, 1997).

Alcohol consumption may contribute significantly to the frequency of injury, through diminished mental faculties and poor judgement (Howland et al., 1996; Blanksby et al., 1997). Young males appear to be more likely to experience spinal injury; in the study by DeVivo & Sekar (1997), 86% of the 341 persons with spinal injuries resulting from swimming pool incidents were men, with an average age of 24 years. A lack of signage may also be a contributory factor. In the same study, almost all the injuries (87%) occurred in private/domestic pools; depth indicators were not present in 75% of cases, and there were no warning signs in 87% of cases (DeVivo & Sekar, 1997).

A proportion of spinal injuries will lead to death by drowning. While data on this are scarce, it does not appear to be common (see, for example, EEA/WHO, 1999). The act of rescue from drowning may also exacerbate spinal cord trauma after the initial impact (Mennen, 1981; Blanksby et al., 1997) because of the movements of the spine during the rescue technique.

2.2.2 Preventive and management actions

The principal contributory factors and preventive actions for spinal cord injuries are summarized in Table 2.3. Evidence suggests that diving technique and education are important in injury prevention (Perrine et al., 1994; Blanksby et al., 1997), and preventive programmes can be effective. In Ontario, for example, the establishment of preventive programmes by Sportsmart Canada and widespread education decreased the incidence of water-related injuries substantially between 1989 and 1992 (Tator et al., 1993).

Because of the young age of many injured persons, awareness raising and education regarding safe behaviours are required early in life. Many countries have school-age swimming instruction that may inadequately stress safe diving, but which may provide a forum for increased public safety (Damjan & Turk, 1995). Education and awareness raising appear to offer the most potential for diving injury prevention, in part because some people have been found to take little notice of posted signs and regulations (Hill, 1984) in isolation.

Table 2.3. Spinal injury: Principal contributory factors and preventive and management actions

Contributory factors

- Diving into a shallow pool or the shallow end of a pool
- Diving into a pool of unknown depth
- Improper diving
- Jumping or diving into water from trees/balconies/other structures
- Poor underwater visibility
- Alcohol consumption
- Lack of supervision
- Lack of signage

Preventive and management actions

- Lifeguard supervision
- General public (user) awareness of depth hazards and safe behaviours
- Early education in diving hazards and safe behaviours/diving instruction
- Restriction of alcohol provision or supervision where alcohol is likely to be consumed
- Poolside wall markings
- Access to emergency services

2.3 Brain and head injuries

Impact on the skull and injuries to the head, including scalp and facial abrasions and breaks, have been associated with swimming pools and similar environments and may result in permanent neurological disability, as well as disfigurement. The contributory factors and preventive and management actions are similar to those for spinal injuries and for limb and minor impact injuries and are summarized in Table 2.3 and Table 2.4.

2.4 Fractures, dislocations, other impact injuries, cuts and lesions

Arm, hand, leg and foot/toe injuries have occurred from a variety of activities in pools and their immediate surroundings. Expert opinion suggests that these incidents are common and generally go unreported. Slippery decks, uneven pavements, uncovered drains and exposed pool spouts may cause injuries to pool users. Reckless water entries, such as jumping onto others in the pool from poolside or from dive boards on the pool deck, jumping into shallow water, running on decks and water slide-related incidents (see Section 2.7), may also result in injury. Slip, trip and fall accidents may be the result of swimming aids, such as rings, floats, etc., left around the pool area. There are reports of injuries sustained as a result of stepping on glass, broken bottles and cans. Banning of glass containers and use of alternative materials for drinks in the pool and hot tub area will minimize these types of injuries.

Maintenance of surfaces, supervision of pool users, providing appropriate warnings, improved pool design and construction, ensuring good underwater visibility and pool safety education are among the actions that can reduce these incidents. Table 2.4 provides examples of some of the factors that contribute to impact injuries and associated preventive and management actions.

Table 2.4. Limb, minor impact injuries, cuts and lesions: Principal contributory factors and preventive and management actions

Contributory factors
• Diving or jumping into shallow water
• Overcrowded pool
• Underwater objects (e.g. ladders)
• Poor underwater visibility
• Slippery decks
• Glass or rubbish around the pool area
• Swimming aids left poolside

Preventive and management actions
• Lifeguard supervision
• General user awareness of hazards and safe behaviours
• Appropriate surface type selection
• Appropriate cleaning and litter control
• Use of alternative materials to glass
• Limits on bather numbers

2.5 Disembowelment

In addition to hair and body entrapment resulting in drowning (Section 2.1.1), there have been reports of incidents in which the suction from the pool or spa drain has pulled intestines out of the body (Hultman & Morgan, 1994; Porter et al., 1997; Gomez-Juarez et al., 2001). In the USA, for example, 18 incidents of evisceration/disembowelment were reported to the CPSC during a 20-year period (CPSC, undated). In the UK, a six-year-old girl suffered a rectal prolapse after being sucked onto a swimming pool drain from which the cover had been removed (Davison & Puntis, 2003). The drain, which was located on the second of the steps giving access to the water, had not been recovered after cleaning.

The drain covers in pools and hot tubs can become brittle and crack, or they may become loose or go missing. If a person sits on a broken cover or uncovered drain, the resulting suction force can cause disembowelment. This is a particular hazard for young children in shallow pools.

Preventive measures are similar to those against entrapment leading to drowning (see Table 2.2). It is uncertain if reduced vacuum (e.g. through multiple outlets and a maximum velocity – see Section 2.1.2) is as effective against disembowelment injuries as it is against drowning, since these occur almost immediately at a small pressure differential. It is recommended that drain covers be designed to avoid the possibility of disembowelment by, for example, having no openings on the top, with the water entering the drain through a series of openings on the side.

2.6 Hazards associated with temperature extremes

Water ranging in temperature from 26 to 30 °C is comfortable for most swimmers throughout prolonged periods of moderate physical exertion. The comfortable upper limit of water temperature for recreational immersion varies from individual to individual and seems to depend on psychological rather than physiological considerations.

Body overheating can occur in natural spas and hot tubs, where water temperatures may be above 40 °C. High temperatures can cause drowsiness, which may lead to unconsciousness (especially when associated with alcohol consumption), resulting in drowning (Press, 1991; see Section 2.1). In addition, high temperatures can lead to heat stroke and death (CPSC, undated). The CPSC has received reports of several deaths from extremely hot water (approximately 43 °C) in hot tubs (CPSC, undated). It is recommended that water temperatures in hot tubs be kept below 40 °C.

Plunge pools present similar problems, but at the other temperature extreme. These small, deep pools generally contain water at a temperature of 8–10 °C and are used in conjunction with saunas or steam baths. Adverse health outcomes that may result from the intense and sudden changes in temperature associated with the use of these pools include immediate impaired coordination, loss of control of breathing and, after some time when the core body temperature has fallen, slowed heart beat, hypothermia, muscle cramps and loss of consciousness.

In general, exposure to temperature extremes should be avoided by pregnant women, users with medical problems and young children, and prolonged immersion in hot tubs or other pools with high or low temperatures should be avoided or approached with caution.

Educational displays and warning signs, warnings from lifeguards and pool staff, regulations on time limits for exposure and limiting use by people with medical conditions are some examples of preventive actions for hazards associated with temperature extremes (see Table 2.5). Further information on this subject is given in Volume 1 of the *Guidelines for Safe Recreational Water Environments* (WHO, 2003).

Table 2.5. Hazards associated with temperature extremes: Principal contributory factors and preventive and management actions

Contributory factors
• Cold plunge when not conditioned • Prolonged immersion in hot water
Preventive and management actions
• Supervision • Signage, including time limits for exposure • A maximum temperature of 40 °C for hot tubs • Gradual immersion • Medical recommendations for pregnant women, people with medical conditions • Limitation of alcohol intake prior to use of hot tubs

2.7 Injuries associated with 'feature pools'

Pools may contain features that present their own particular requirements to ensure safe use. Water slides add excitement but may present physical hazards, particularly where riders go down in pairs, too close to each other or headfirst; or where riders stop, slow down or stand up on the slide. Failure to leave the area immediately after arriving from the slide may also present physical hazards. In the USA, CDC reported injuries relating to the use of a water slide (CDC, 1984). The slide consisted of two fibreglass tubes, 1.2 m wide and over 100 m in length. In a six-week period, 65 people were injured while using the slide and sought medical care. Injuries included fractures, concussions, bruises and abrasions and sprains and strains. This included nine spinal fractures.

Wave machines may provide a higher level of excitement and also often increased bather load. Extra vigilance is needed by lifeguards and bathers alike. The possibility exists for entrapment of limbs in wave machine chambers; therefore, all parts of the wave machine should be enclosed by a guard. As grilles must be large enough to allow water flow, adequate supervision to prevent users holding onto the grilles, when the waves are in action, may also be necessary.

In-water features may also present a physical hazard, as they may be slippery or encourage climbing, falls from which could injure the climber or other user. Design issues, user awareness and education are important considerations in feature pools.

2.8 References

Asher KN, Rivara FP, Felix D, Vance L, Dunne R (1995) Water safety training as a potential means of reducing risk of young children's drowning. *Injury Prevention*, 1(4): 228–233.

Bierens JJLM (1996) 2944 submersion victims: an analysis of external causes, concomitant risk factors, complications and prognosis. In: *Drownings in the Netherlands. Pathophysiology, epidemiology and clinical studies*, PhD thesis Netherlands, University of Utrecht.

Blanksby BA, Wearne FK, Elliott BC, Biltvich JD (1997) Aetiology and occurrence of diving injuries. A review of diving safety. *Sports Medicine*, 23(4): 228–246.

Blum C, Shield J (2000) Toddler drowning in domestic swimming pools. *Injury Prevention*, 6: 288–290.

Branche CM, Sniezek JE, Sattin RW, Mirkin IR (1991) Water recreation-related spinal injuries: Risk factors in natural bodies of water. *Accident Analysis and Prevention*, 23(1): 13–17.

Brenner R (2005) Swimming lessons, swimming ability and the risk of drowning. In: Bierens JJLM et al., eds. *Handbook on drowning. Prevention, rescue and treatment*. Netherlands, Springer, in press.

Browne Ml, Lewis-Michl EL, Stark AD (2003) Unintentional drownings among New York State residents, 1988–1994. *Public Health Reports*, 118(5): 448–458.

CDC (1984) Injuries at a water slide – Washington. *Morbidity and Mortality Weekly Report*, 33(27): 379–382, 387.

CDC (1990) Current trends child drownings and near drownings associated with swimming pools – Maricopa County, Arizona, 1988 and 1989. *Morbidity and Mortality Weekly Report*, 39(26): 441–442.

CDC (2004) Nonfatal and fatal drownings in recreational water settings – United States, 2001–2002. *Morbidity and Mortality Weekly Report*, 53(21): 447–452.

CPSC (undated) *Spas, hot tubs, and whirlpools*. Washington, DC, United States Consumer Product Safety Commission (CPSC Document #5112; http://www.cpsc.gov/cpscpub/pubs/5112.html, accessed 15 November 2004).

Craig AB Jr (1976) Summary of 58 cases of loss of consciousness during underwater swimming and diving. *Medicine and Science in Sports*, 8(3): 171–175.

Cummings P, Quan L (1999) Trends in unintentional drowning. The role of alcohol and medical care. *Journal of the American Medical Association*, 281: 2198–2202.

Damjan H, Turk KK (1995) Prevention of spinal injuries from diving in Slovenia. *Paraplegia*, 33(5): 246–249.

Davison A, Puntis JWL (2003) Awareness of swimming pool suction injury among tour operators. *Archives of Diseases in Childhood*, 88: 584–586.

DeVivo MJ, Sekar P (1997) Prevention of spinal cord injuries that occur in swimming pools. *Spinal Cord*, 35(8): 509–515.

Dietz PE, Baker SP (1974) Drowning. Epidemiology and prevention. *American Journal of Public Health*, 64(4): 303–312.

EEA/WHO (1999) *Water resources and human health in Europe*. European Environment Agency and World Health Organization Regional Office for Europe.

Gabrielsen JL, ed. (1988) *Diving safety: a position paper*. Indianapolis, IN, United States Diving.

Gomez-Juarez M, Cascales P, Garcia-Olmo D, Gomez-Juarez F, Usero S, Capilla P, Garcia-Blazquez E, Anderica F (2001) Complete evisceration of the small intestine through a perianal wound as a result of suction at a wading pool. *Journal of Trauma*, 51: 398–399.

Hill V (1984) History of diving accidents. In: *Proceedings of the New South Wales Symposium on Water Safety*. Sydney, New South Wales, Department of Sport and Recreation, pp. 28–33.

Howland J, Hingson R (1988) Alcohol as a risk factor for drowning: a review of the literature (1950–1985). *Accident Analysis and Prevention*, 20: 19–25.

Howland J, Hingson R, Mangione TW, Bell N, Bak S (1996) Why are most drowning victims men? Sex difference in aquatic skills and behaviours. *American Journal of Public Health*, 86(1): 93–96.

Hultman CS, Morgan R (1994) Transanal intestinal evisceration following suction from an uncovered swimming pool drain: case report. *Journal of Trauma*, 37(5): 843–847.

Kyriacou DN, Arcinue EL, Peek C, Kraus JF (1994) Effect of immediate resuscitation on children with submersion injury. *Pediatrics*, 94: 137–142.

Levin DL, Morris FC, Toro LO, Brink LW, Turner G (1993) Drowning and near-drowning. *Pediatric Clinics in North America*, 40: 321–336.

Liller KD, Kent AB, Arcari C, MacDermott RJ (1993) Risk factors for drowning and near-drowning among children in Hillsborough County, Florida. *Public Health Reports*, 108(3): 346–353.

Mackie I (1978) Alcohol and aquatic disasters. *Medical Journal of Australia*, 1(12): 652–653.

Mackie I (2005) Availability and quality of data to assess the global burden of drowning. In: Bierens JJLM et al., eds. *Handbook on drowning. Prevention, rescue and treatment*. Netherlands, Springer, in press.

Mennen U (1981) A survey of spinal injuries from diving. A study of patients in Pretoria and Cape Town. *South African Medical Journal*, 59(22): 788–790.

Milliner N, Pearn J, Guard R (1980) Will fenced pools save lives? A 10-year study from Mulgrave Shire, Queensland. *Medical Journal of Australia*, 2: 510–511.

Minaire P, Demolin P, Bourret J, Girard R, Berard E, Deidier C, Eyssette M, Biron A (1983) Life expectancy following spinal cord injury: a ten-years survey in the Rhone-Alpes Region, France, 1969–1980. *Paraplegia*, 21(1): 11–15.

National Center for Health Statistics (1998) *National mortality data, 1997*. Hyattsville, MD, Centers for Disease Control and Prevention.

Nichter MA, Everett PB (1989) Childhood near-drowning: is cardiopulmonary resuscitation always indicated? *Critical Care Medicine*, 17(10): 993–995.

Orlowski JP (1989) It's time for pediatricians to "rally round the pool fence". *Pediatrics*, 83: 1065–1066.

Patetta MJ, Biddinger PW (1988) Characteristics of drowning deaths in North Carolina. *Public Health Reports*, 103(4): 406–411.

Pearn J, Nixon J (1977) Prevention of childhood drowning accidents. *Medical Journal of Australia*, 1(17): 616–618.

Pearn J, Nixon J, Wilkey I (1976) Freshwater drowning and near-drowning accidents involving children: A five-year total population study. *Medical Journal of Australia*, 2(25–26): 942–946.

Peden M, McGee K (2003) The epidemiology of drowning worldwide. *Injury Control and Safety Promotion*, 10(4): 195–199.

Pepe P, Bierens J (2005) Resuscitation: an overview. In: Bierens JJLM et al., eds. *Handbook on drowning. Prevention, rescue and treatment*. Netherlands, Springer, in press.

Perrine MW, Mundt JC, Weiner RI (1994) When alcohol and water don't mix: diving under the influence. *Journal of Studies on Alcohol*, 55(5): 517–524.

Petridou E (2005) Risk factors for drowning and near-drowning injuries. In: Bierens JJLM et al., eds. *Handbook on drowning. Prevention, rescue and treatment*. Netherlands, Springer, in press.

Plueckhahn VD (1979) Drowning: community aspects. *Medical Journal of Australia*, 2(5): 226–228.

Porter ES, Kohlstadt IC, Farrell KP (1997) Preventing wading pool suction-drain injuries. *Maryland Medical Journal*, 46(6): 297–298.

Present P (1987) *Child drowning study: A report on the epidemiology of drowning in residential pools to children under age 5*. Washington, DC, United States Consumer Product Safety Commission, Directorate for Epidemiology.

Press E (1991) The health hazards of saunas and spas and how to minimize them. *American Journal of Public Health*, 81(8): 1034–1037.

Quan L, Gore EJ, Wentz K, Allen J, Novack AH (1989) Ten year study of pediatric drownings and near drownings in King County, Washington: lessons in injury prevention. *Pediatrics*, 83(6): 1035–1040.

Ryan CA, Dowling G (1993) Drowning deaths in people with epilepsy. *Canadian Medical Association Journal*, 148(3): 270.

Sibert JR, Lyons RA, Smith BA, Cornall P, Sumner V, Craven MA, Kemp AM on behalf of the Safe Water Information Monitor Collaboration (2002) Preventing deaths by drowning in children in the United Kingdom: have we made progress in 10 years? Population based incidence study. *British Medical Journal*, 324: 1070–1071.

Smith GS (2005) The global burden of drowning. In: Bierens JJLM et al., eds. *Handbook on drowning. Prevention, rescue and treatment*. Netherlands, Springer, in press.

Spyker DA (1985) Submersion injury. Epidemiology, prevention and management. *Pediatric Clinics of North America*, 32(1): 113–125.

Steinbruck K, Paeslack V (1980) Analysis of 139 spinal cord injuries due to accidents in water sport. *Paraplegia*, 18(2): 86–93.

Stevenson MR, Rimajova M, Edgecombe D, Vickery K (2003) Childhood drowning: barriers surrounding private swimming pools. *Pediatrics*, 111(2): e115–e119.

Stover SL, Fine PR (1987) The epidemiology and economics of spinal cord injury. *Paraplegia*, 25(3): 225–228.

Tator CH, Edmonds VE (1986) Sports and recreation are a rising cause of spinal cord injury. *Physician and Sportsmedicine*, 14: 157–167.

Tator CH, Edmonds VE, Lapeczak X (1993) *Ontario Catastrophic Sports Recreational Injuries Survey. July 1, 1991 – July 30, 1992*. Toronto, Ontario, Think First Canada.

Think First Foundation (2004) Think First Foundation website (http://www.thinkfirst.org/news/facts.html), accessed 2 March 2004.

Thompson DC, Rivara FP (2000) Pool fencing for preventing drowning in children. *Cochrane Database of Systematic Reviews*, 2: CD001047.

WHO (2003) *Guidelines for safe recreational water environments. Vol. 1: Coastal and fresh waters*. Geneva, World Health Organization.

WHO (2004) *The World Health Report 2004: Changing history*. Geneva, World Health Organization.

Wintemute GJ, Kraus JF, Teret SP, Wright M (1987) Drowning in childhood and adolescence: a population-based study. *American Journal of Public Health*, 77: 830–832.

World Congress on Drowning (2002) Recommendations. In: *Proceedings of the World Congress on Drowning*. Amsterdam, 26–28 June 2002.

Yanai T, Hay JG, Gerot JT (1996) Three dimensional videography of swimming with panning periscopes. *Journal of Biomechanics*, 33(5): 246–249.

CHAPTER 3
Microbial hazards

A variety of microorganisms can be found in swimming pools and similar recreational water environments, which may be introduced in a number of ways.

In many cases, the risk of illness or infection has been linked to faecal contamination of the water. The faecal contamination may be due to faeces released by bathers or a contaminated source water or, in outdoor pools, may be the result of direct animal contamination (e.g. from birds and rodents). Faecal matter is introduced into the water when a person has an accidental faecal release – AFR (through the release of formed stool or diarrhoea into the water) or residual faecal material on swimmers' bodies is washed into the pool (CDC, 2001a). Many of the outbreaks related to swimming pools would have been prevented or reduced if the pool had been well managed.

Non-faecal human shedding (e.g. from vomit, mucus, saliva or skin) in the swimming pool or similar recreational water environments is a potential source of pathogenic organisms. Infected users can directly contaminate pool or hot tub waters and the surfaces of objects or materials at a facility with pathogens (notably viruses or fungi), which may lead to skin infections in other patrons who come in contact with the contaminated water or surfaces. 'Opportunistic pathogens' (notably bacteria) can also be shed from users and transmitted via surfaces and contaminated water.

Some bacteria, most notably non-faecally-derived bacteria (see Section 3.4), may accumulate in biofilms and present an infection hazard. In addition, certain free-living aquatic bacteria and amoebae can grow in pool, natural spa or hot tub waters, in pool or hot tub components or facilities (including heating, ventilation and air-conditioning [HVAC] systems) or on other wet surfaces within the facility to a point at which some of them may cause a variety of respiratory, dermal or central nervous system infections or diseases. Outdoor pools may also be subject to microorganisms derived directly from pets and wildlife.

This chapter describes illness and infection associated with microbial contamination of swimming pools, natural spas and hot tubs. The sections reflect the origin of the microbial contaminant, as illustrated in Figure 3.1. In each case, a short subsection on risk assessment and risk management is given, although general management strategies for managing air and water quality are described in detail in Chapter 5.

In most cases, monitoring for potential microbial hazards is done using indicator microorganisms (rather than specific microbial pathogens), which are easy to enumerate and would be expected to be present in greater numbers than pathogens. The traditional role of indicator parameters was to show the presence or absence of faecal pollution in water supplies. The criteria associated with microbial indicators of pollution are outlined in Box 3.1 and further discussed in WHO (2004). The use of these microorganisms in monitoring water quality is covered in Chapter 5.

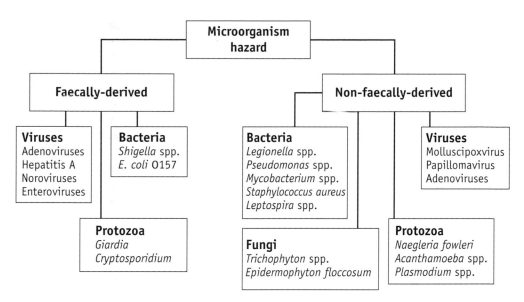

Figure 3.1. Potential microbial hazards in pools and similar environments

BOX 3.1 CRITERIA FOR INDICATOR ORGANISMS AND THEIR APPLICATION TO POOLS AND SIMILAR ENVIRONMENTS

- The indicator should be absent in unpolluted environments and present when the source of pathogenic microorganisms of concern is present (e.g. faecal material).
- The indicator should not multiply in the environment.
- The indicator should be present in greater numbers than the pathogenic microorganisms.
- The indicator should respond to natural environmental conditions and water treatment processes in a manner similar to the pathogens of concern.
- The indicator should be easy to isolate, identify and enumerate.
- Indicator tests should be inexpensive, thereby permitting numerous samples to be taken (if appropriate).

Microorganisms that are used to assess the microbial quality of swimming pool and similar environments include heterotrophic plate count – HPC (a general measure of non-specific microbial levels), faecal indicators (such as thermotolerant coliforms, *E. coli*), *Pseudomonas aeruginosa*, *Staphylococcus aureus* and *Legionella* spp. HPC, thermotolerant coliforms and *E. coli* are indicators in the strict sense of the definition.

As health risks in pools and similar environments may be faecal or non-faecal in origin, both faecal indicators and non-faecally-derived microorganisms (e.g. *P. aeruginosa*, *S. aureus* and *Legionella* spp.) should be examined. Faecal indicators are used to monitor for the possible presence of faecal contamination; HPC, *Pseudomonas aeruginosa* and *Legionella* spp. can be used to examine growth, and *Staphylococcus aureus* can be used to determine non-faecal shedding. The absence of these organisms, however, does not guarantee safety, as some pathogens are more resistant to treatment than the indicators, and there is no perfect indicator organism.

3.1 Faecally-derived viruses

3.1.1 Hazard identification

The viruses that have been linked to swimming pool outbreaks are shown in Table 3.1. Viruses cannot multiply in water, and therefore their presence must be a consequence of pollution. Some adenoviruses may also be shed from eyes and the throat and are responsible for swimming pool conjunctivitis.

Viruses of six types (rotavirus, norovirus, adenovirus, astrovirus, enterovirus and hepatitis A virus) are all shed following infection. Clinical data show that rotaviruses are by far the most prevalent cause of viral gastroenteritis in children, and noroviruses cause the most cases of viral diarrhoea in adults. However, few waterborne pool outbreaks have been associated with these agents. Although outbreaks are highlighted, it should be kept in mind that non-outbreak disease is likely to occur and that virus-associated pool or hot tub outbreaks are very uncommon. Even when outbreaks are detected, the evidence linking the outbreak to the pool is generally circumstantial. In the outbreaks summarized in Table 3.1, the etiological agents were detected in the water in only two cases (D'Angelo et al., 1979; Papapetropoulou & Vantarakis, 1998).

3.1.2 Outbreaks of viral illness associated with pools

1. Adenovirus-related outbreaks

There are over 50 types of adenoviruses (Hunter, 1997), and while some may cause enteric infections and are therefore shed in faeces, they are also associated with respiratory and ocular symptoms and non-faecally-derived transmission. Types 40 and 41 cause gastroenteritis in young children, but there is no documented association with waterborne transmission.

Foy et al. (1968) reported an outbreak of pharyngo-conjunctival fever caused by adenovirus type 3. The infection occurred in two children's swimming teams after exposure to unchlorinated swimming pool water. The attack rates in the two teams were 65% and 67%, respectively. The main symptoms were fever, pharyngitis and conjunctivitis. The virus could not be isolated from the pool water. The authors speculated that faecal contamination of the unchlorinated swimming pool water could have been the source of the contamination.

Caldwell et al. (1974) reported an outbreak of conjunctivitis associated with adenovirus type 7 in seven members of a community swimming team. The main symptoms were associated with the eyes. An investigation of the pool-related facilities suggested that the school swimming pool was the source of the infection, as both the pool chlorinator and pool filter had failed. The outbreak was brought under control by raising the pool's free residual chlorine level above 0.3 mg/l.

Adenovirus type 4 was the causative agent of a swimming pool-related outbreak of pharyngo-conjunctivitis reported by D'Angelo et al. (1979). A total of 72 cases were identified. Adenovirus type 4 was isolated from 20 of 26 swab specimens. The virus was also detected in samples of pool water. An investigation showed that inadequate levels of chlorine had been added to the pool water, resulting in no free chlorine in pool water samples. Adequate chlorination and closing the pool for the summer stopped the outbreak of illness.

Table 3.1. Summary of waterborne disease outbreaks associated with pools due to faecally-excreted viruses

Etiological agent	Source of agent	Disinfection/ treatment	Reference
Adenovirus 3	Possible faecal contamination	None	Foy et al., 1968
Adenovirus 7	Unknown	Improper chlorination	Caldwell et al., 1974
Adenovirus 4	Unknown	Inadequate chlorine level	D'Angelo et al., 1979
Adenovirus 3	Unknown	Pool filter system defect, failed chlorinator	Martone et al., 1980
Adenovirus 7a	Unknown	Malfunctioning chlorinator	Turner et al., 1987
Adenoviruses	Unknown	Inadequate chlorination	Papapetropoulou & Vantarakis, 1998
Adenovirus 3	Unknown	Inadequate chlorination and pool maintenance	Harley et al., 2001
Hepatitis A	Accidental faecal release suspected	None	Solt et al., 1994
	Cross-connection to sewer line	Operating properly	Mahoney et al., 1992
Norovirus	Unknown	Chlorinator disconnected	Kappus et al., 1982
	Probably via public toilets	Manual chlorination three times a week	Maunula et al., 2004
	No details available	No details available	Yoder et al., 2004
	No details available	No details available	Yoder et al., 2004
	Possible faecal contamination	Chlorination failure	CDC, 2004
Echovirus 30	Vomit	Operating properly	Kee et al., 1994

A second outbreak in the same locality and year was linked to adenovirus type 3 and swimming activity (Martone et al., 1980). Based on surveys, at least 105 cases were identified. The illness was characterized by sore throat, fever, headache and anorexia. Conjunctivitis affected only 34 of the individuals. Use of a swimming pool was linked to the illness. The outbreak coincided with a temporary defect in the pool filter system and probably improper maintenance of chlorine levels. The authors suspected that the level of free chlorine in the pool water was less than 0.4 mg/l. They also pointed out that while the virus was probably transmitted through water, person-to-person transmission could not be ruled out.

In 1987, an outbreak of adenovirus type 7a infection was associated with a swimming pool (Turner et al., 1987). Seventy-seven individuals were identified with the symptoms of pharyngitis (inflammation of the pharynx). A telephone survey indicated that persons who swam at the community swimming pool were more likely to be ill than those who did not. Swimmers who reported swallowing water were more likely to be ill than those who did not. Further investigation showed that the pool chlorinator had reportedly malfunctioned during the period when the outbreak occurred. The outbreak ceased when proper chlorination was reinstated.

An outbreak of pharyngo-conjunctivitis caused by adenoviruses occurred among swimmers participating in a competition. Over 80 people were found to be suffering from symptoms. Adenoviruses were identified in swimming pool samples using nested polymerase chain reaction, and poor chlorination (residual chlorine levels <0.2 mg/l) was considered to have contributed to the outbreak (Papapetropoulou & Vantarakis, 1998).

In 2000, an outbreak of illness related to adenovirus type 3 was detected. It was found that there was a strong association between the presence of symptoms and swimming at a school camp. Although adenoviruses were not isolated from the pool water, inspection of the pool revealed that it was poorly maintained and inadequately chlorinated (Harley et al., 2001).

2. Hepatitis A-related outbreaks

Solt et al. (1994) reported an outbreak in Hungary in which 31 children were hospitalized following hepatitis A infection. Investigation of potential common sources eliminated food, drink and person-to-person transmission. All of the patients had reported swimming at a summer camp swimming pool. Further investigation discovered 25 additional cases. All of the cases were males between the ages of 5 and 17 years. The pool, which was not chlorinated, was half full of water for a period and was used by younger children. The pool was generally overcrowded during the month of August. It was concluded that the crowded conditions and generally poor hygienic conditions contributed to the outbreak.

An outbreak of hepatitis A in several states in the USA during 1989, which may have been associated with a public swimming pool, was reported by Mahoney et al. (1992). Twenty of 822 campers developed hepatitis A infections. Case–control studies indicated that swimmers or those who used a specific hot tub were more likely than controls to become ill. It was hypothesized that a cross-connection between a sewage line and the pool water intake line may have been responsible for the outbreak or that one of the swimmers may have contaminated the water. The disinfectant levels in the pools met local standards.

3. Norovirus-related outbreaks

Few outbreaks of norovirus-related disease (previously known as Norwalk virus or Norwalk-like viruses) associated with swimming pools have been reported. Kappus et al. (1982) reported an outbreak of norovirus gastroenteritis associated with a swimming pool that affected 103 individuals. The illness typically lasted 24 h and was characterized by vomiting and cramping. Serological studies suggested that norovirus was the cause of the gastroenteritis among the swimmers. Case–control studies indicated that swimmers were more likely than non-swimmers to become ill. Similarly, the attack rate was significantly higher in swimmers who had swallowed water than in those who had not. The pool chlorinator had not been reconnected before the outbreak, which occurred at the beginning of the swimming season. The source of the virus was not found.

Maunula et al. (2004) reported an outbreak of gastroenteritis associated with norovirus contracted from a wading pool in Helsinki, Finland. Norovirus and astrovirus were isolated from water samples taken from the pool. The pool was heavily used during the summer months (with as many as 500 bathers a day) and was manually chlorinated three times a week. There was no routine monitoring of free chlorine. It is believed that the pool had been heavily contaminated with human faecal material, with the contamination apparently being carried from the public toilets, situated very close to the pool, which were found to be grossly contaminated (although a number of nappies were also found at the bottom of the pool during the cleaning operation). The pool was emptied and cleaned and subsequently fitted with continuous filtration and chlorination.

Yoder et al. (2004) reported two outbreaks of norovirus infection that were associated with swimming pools in the USA between 2000 and 2002, one of which was associated with a hotel pool and hot tub, but gave no other details.

CDC (2004) reported an outbreak of gastroenteritis in children, whose only common exposure was attendance at a swimming club the previous weekend. Fifty-three people reported illness, and norovirus was isolated from a number of cases. An undetected accidental faecal release was suspected, and poor pool water quality monitoring and maintenance contributed to the outbreak.

4. Enterovirus-related outbreaks

Enteroviruses include polioviruses, echoviruses and coxsackieviruses types A and B. The only documented case of enterovirus infection following pool exposure was associated with echovirus, as reported by Kee et al. (1994). Thirty-three bathers had symptoms of vomiting, diarrhoea and headache shortly after swimming in an outdoor swimming pool. The outbreak is believed to have been caused by a bather who swam while ill and vomited into the pool. Individuals who had swallowed water were more likely to become ill than those who had not. Echovirus 30 was isolated from the case who had vomited and from six other cases. Proper disinfectant levels had been maintained at the pool, but they were inadequate to contain the risk of infection from vomit in the pool water.

3.1.3 Risk assessment

Determination of polluted pool water as the unequivocal cause of a viral disease outbreak requires the detection of the virus in a water sample. This is clearly not a routine procedure, but is something that is done in response to a suspected disease outbreak. Concentration techniques for viruses in water are available (e.g. SCA, 1995 and reviewed by Wyn-Jones & Sellwood, 2001), which may be adapted to pool water samples. Some agents (e.g. enteroviruses) may be detected in cell culture, but most (e.g. adenoviruses 40 and 41 and noroviruses) require molecular detection methods. If the virus has remained in contact with water containing free disinfectant for some time, then detection of infectious virus may not be possible.

Enteric viruses occur in high numbers in the faeces of infected individuals. Hepatitis A virus has been found at densities of 10^{10} per gram (Coulepis et al., 1980), and noroviruses have been estimated at 10^{11} per gram, although echoviruses may reach only 10^6 per gram. Given the high densities at which some viruses can be shed by infected individuals, it is not surprising that accidental faecal releases into swimming pools and hot tubs can lead to high attack rates in pools where outbreaks occur, especially if the faecal release is undetected or detected but not responded to adequately.

1. *Adenoviruses*

   Most adenoviruses can be grown in commonly available cell cultures, with the exception of types 40 and 41, which may be detected by molecular biological techniques, principally by the polymerase chain reaction – PCR (Kidd et al., 1996). Types 40 and 41 are those usually associated with gastroenteritis. Other types, though more usually associated with infections of the eyelids and/or throat (pharyngo-conjunctival fever), may also be shed in the faeces for extended periods (Fox et al., 1969). The attack rate for swimming pool outbreaks linked to adenovirus serotypes is moderately high, ranging from 18% to 52% (Martone et al., 1980; Turner et al., 1987).

2. *Hepatitis A virus*

   Culture of hepatitis A virus is generally impractical, and detection relies on molecular methods (reverse transcriptase polymerase chain reaction – RT-PCR). The virus is transmitted by the faecal–oral route, with water and sewage being a frequent source of infection. The disease has an incubation period of 15–50 days, anorexia, nausea, vomiting and often jaundice being the common symptoms. Virus is shed before the onset of symptoms. The attack rate in one outbreak of illness associated with a swimming pool ranged from 1.2% to 6.1% in swimmers less than 18 years of age (Mahoney et al., 1992).

3. *Noroviruses*

   Environmental detection of these agents is restricted to RT-PCR since there is no cell culture system available. Symptoms occur within 48 h of exposure and include diarrhoea, vomiting, nausea and fever. Virus shedding, as detected by electron microscopy, stops soon after onset of symptoms, but is detectable by RT-PCR for up to five days. Attack rates are generally very high; Kappus et al. (1982), for example, reported an attack rate of 71% for those swimmers who had swallowed water.

4. *Enteroviruses*

   Coxsackieviruses are frequently found in polluted waters, and vaccine poliovirus is also found where there is a high percentage of individuals immunized (although no investigations have been reported where this has been found in pool water). Echoviruses are found less often. None of the enteroviruses commonly cause gastroenteritis in the absence of other disease, and, although they are associated with a wide variety of symptoms, most infections are asymptomatic.

3.1.4 *Risk management*

The control of viruses in swimming pool water and similar environments is usually accomplished by proper treatment, including the application of disinfectants. Episodes of gross contamination of a swimming pool due to an accidental faecal release or vomit from an infected person cannot be effectively controlled by normal disinfectant levels. The only approach to maintaining public health protection under conditions of an accidental faecal release or vomit is to prevent the use of the pool until the contaminants are inactivated (see Chapter 5). The education of parents/caregivers of small children and other water users about good hygienic behaviour at swimming pools is another approach that may prove to be useful for improving health safety at swimming pools and the reduction of accidental faecal releases. It is recommended that people with gastroenteritis should not use public or semi-public pools and hot tubs while ill or for at least a week after their illness, in order to avoid transmitting the illness to other pool or hot tub users.

3.2 Faecally-derived bacteria

3.2.1 Hazard identification

Shigella species and *Escherichia coli* O157 are two related bacteria that have been linked to outbreaks of illness associated with swimming in pools or similar environments. *Shigella* has been responsible for outbreaks related to artificial ponds and other small bodies of water where water movement has been very limited. The lack of water movement means that these water bodies behave very much as if they were swimming pools, except that chlorination or other forms of disinfection are not being used. Similar non-pool outbreaks have been described for *E. coli* O157, although there have also been two outbreaks reported where the source was a children's paddling pool. These outbreaks are summarized in Table 3.2, as they illustrate the potential risk that might be experienced in swimming pools under similar conditions, although only the pool specific outbreaks are covered in detail.

3.2.2 Outbreaks of bacterial illness associated with pools

1. Shigella-related outbreaks

An outbreak of shigellosis associated with a fill-and-drain wading pool (filled on a daily basis with potable water) was reported from Iowa, USA (CDC, 2001b). The pool, which had a maximum depth of 35 cm, was frequented by very young and non-toilet-trained children. The pool had neither recirculation nor disinfection. One pool sample was found to contain thermotolerant coliforms and *E. coli*. Sixty-nine people were considered to be infected with shigellosis, of which 26 cases were laboratory confirmed as *S. sonnei*. It is thought that the transmission of shigellosis over several days may have been a result of residual contaminated water present after draining and people with diarrhoea visiting the pool on subsequent days.

2. E. coli O157-related outbreaks

In 1992, an outbreak of *E. coli* O157 infection was epidemiologically and clinically linked to a collapsible children's paddling pool (Brewster et al., 1994). Six cases of diarrhoea, including one case of haemolytic uraemic syndrome, and one asymptomatic case were identified. *E. coli* O157 phage type 59 was isolated from the six cases. The pool had not been drained or disinfected over the three-day period surrounding the outbreak. It was believed that the pool had been initially contaminated by a child known to have diarrhoea.

In 1993, six children with haemorrhagic colitis, three of whom developed haemolytic uraemic syndrome, were epidemiologically linked to a disinfected public paddling pool (Hildebrand et al., 1996). *E. coli* O157 phage type 2 was isolated from faecal specimens of five cases. *E. coli* (but not *E. coli* O157) was detected in the pool during the investigation. Free chlorine levels in the pool were less than 1 mg/l at the time of sampling.

Table 3.2. Summary of outbreaks of disease associated with pools due to faecally-excreted bacteria

Etiological agent	Source of agent	Disinfection/ treatment	Reference
Shigella spp.	AFR	None	Sorvillo et al., 1988
	Not known	None	Makintubee et al., 1987
	AFR	None	Blostein, 1991
	Likely AFR	None	CDC, 2001b
E. coli O157	AFR	None	Keene et al., 1994
	AFR	Not known	Brewster et al., 1994
	AFR	Inadequate treatment	Hildebrand et al., 1996
	Not known	None	CDC, 1996
	Not known	None	Cransberg et al., 1996

AFR – Accidental faecal release

3.2.3 Risk assessment

Shigella species are small, non-motile, Gram-negative, facultatively anaerobic rods. They ferment glucose but not lactose, with the production of acid but not gas. Symptoms associated with shigellosis include diarrhoea, fever and nausea. The incubation period for shigellosis is 1–3 days. The infection usually lasts for 4–7 days and is self-limiting.

E. coli O157 are small, motile, non-spore-forming, Gram-negative, facultatively anaerobic rods. They ferment glucose and lactose. Unlike most *E. coli*, *E. coli* O157 does not produce glucuronidase, nor does it grow well at 44.5 °C. *E. coli* O157 causes non-bloody diarrhoea, which can progress to bloody diarrhoea and haemolytic uraemic syndrome. Other symptoms include vomiting and fever in more severe cases. The usual incubation period is 3–4 days, but longer periods are not uncommon. In most instances, the illness typically resolves itself in about a week. About 5–10% of individuals develop haemolytic uraemic syndrome following an *E. coli* O157 infection. Haemolytic uraemic syndrome, characterized by haemolytic anaemia and acute renal failure, occurs most frequently in infants, young children and elderly people.

Individuals infected with *E. coli* O157 shed these bacteria at similar or slightly higher densities than the non-enterohaemorrhagic *Shigella*. Literature reports indicate that *E. coli* O157 is known to be shed at densities as high as 10^8 per gram. *Shigella* species are shed at similar but somewhat lower levels by individuals who have contracted shigellosis (Table 3.3).

Table 3.3. Bacterial exposure factors

Agent	Density shed during infection	Duration of shedding	Infective dose	Reference
Shigella	10^6 per gram	30 days	$<5 \times 10^2/ID_{50}$	Makintubee et al., 1987; DuPont, 1988
Escherichia coli O157	10^8 per gram	7–13 days	Not known[a]	Pai et al., 1984

ID_{50} – dose of microorganisms required to infect 50% of individuals exposed
[a] Probably similar to *Shigella*

The infective dose for *Shigella* species is usually between 10 and 100 organisms (Table 3.3). Lower doses, however, may cause illness in infants, the elderly or immunocompromised individuals. The infective dose for *E. coli* O157 is unknown but is likely to be similar to that for *Shigella* species. Keene et al. (1994) suggested that the infective dose is very low, based on experience in an outbreak.

3.2.4 Risk management

One of the primary risk management interventions is to reduce accidental faecal release occurrence in the first place – for example, by educating pool users. *E. coli* O157 and *Shigella* species are readily controlled by chlorine and other disinfectants under ideal conditions. However, if an accidental faecal release has occurred in a swimming pool or hot tub, it is likely that these organisms will not be instantly eliminated, and other steps will have to be taken to provide time for disinfectant effect, such as evacuation of the pool (see Chapter 5).

3.3 Faecally-derived protozoa

3.3.1 Hazard identification

Giardia and particularly *Cryptosporidium* spp. are faecally-derived protozoa that have been linked to outbreaks of illness in swimming pools and similar environments. These two organisms are similar in a number of respects. They have a cyst or oocyst form that is highly resistant to both environmental stress and disinfectants, they have a low infective dose and they are shed in high densities by infected individuals. There have been a number of outbreaks of disease attributed to these pathogens, as summarized in Table 3.4.

3.3.2 Outbreaks of protozoan illness associated with pools

1. Giardia-related outbreaks

Giardiasis has been associated with swimming pools and water slides. In 1994, a case–control study was conducted in the United Kingdom to determine the risk factors for giardiasis. Giardiasis cases were identified from disease surveillance reports over a one-year period (Gray et al., 1994). Seventy-four cases and 108 matched controls were identified. Analysis of the data indicated that swimming appeared to be an independent risk factor for giardiasis. Other recreational exposures and ingestion of potentially contaminated water were found to be not significantly related to giardiasis.

In 1984, a case of giardiasis was reported in a child who had participated in an infant and toddler swim class in Washington State, USA (Harter et al., 1984). The identification of this case of giardiasis led to a stool survey of 70 of the class participants. The stool survey revealed a 61% prevalence of *Giardia* infection. None of the non-swimming playmates was positive. Eight of 23 children (35%) exposed only at a better maintained pool to which the classes had been moved four weeks prior to the survey were positive. The investigators did not find any evidence of transmission to non-swim-class pool users. Adequate chlorine levels were maintained in the pool. Contamination of the pool was thought to be due to an undetected accidental faecal release.

Table 3.4. Summary of disease outbreaks associated with pools due to faecally-derived protozoa

Etiological agent	Source of agent	Disinfection/ treatment	Reference
Giardia	AFR	Inadequate treatment	Harter et al., 1984
	AFR	Inadequate treatment	Porter et al., 1988
	AFR	Adequate treatment	Greensmith et al., 1988
Cryptosporidium	AFR	Adequate treatment	CDC, 1990
	Sewage intrusion	Plumbing defects	Joce et al., 1991
	AFR	Not known	Bell et al., 1993
	Sewage intrusion	Not known	McAnulty et al., 1994
	Not known	Not known	CDC, 1994
	AFR	Adequate treatment	Hunt et al., 1994
	AFR	Adequate treatment	CDSC, 1995
	Likely AFR	Adequate treatment	Sundkist et al., 1997
	AFR	Faulty ozone generator	CDSC, 1997
	Not known	Plumbing and treatment defects	CDSC, 1998
	Not known	Adequate treatment	CDSC, 1999
	Likely AFR	Treatment problems	CDSC, 1999
	Suspected AFR	Adequate treatment	CDSC, 2000
	Likely AFR	Inadequate treatment	CDSC, 2000
	Not known	Adequate treatment	CDSC, 2000
	Not known	Adequate treatment	CDSC, 2000
	Not known	Not known	CDSC, 2000
	Not known	Ozonation problems	CDSC, 2000
	AFR	Not known	CDC, 2001c
	Not known	Not known	Galmes et al., 2003

AFR – accidental faecal release
Adequate treatment – in terms of indicator bacteria monitoring results

In the autumn of 1985, an outbreak of giardiasis occurred among several swimming groups at an indoor pool in north-east New Jersey, USA (Porter et al., 1988). Nine clinical cases were identified, eight of whom had *Giardia*-positive stool specimens. All were female, seven were adults (>18 years), and two were children. A 39% attack rate was observed for the group of women who had exposure on one day. These cases had no direct contact with children or other risk factors for acquiring *Giardia*. Infection most likely occurred following ingestion of swimming pool water contaminated with *Giardia* cysts. The source of *Giardia* contamination was a child who had a faecal accident in the pool, who was a member of the group that swam the same day as the women's swimming group. A stool survey of the child's group showed that of 20 people tested, 8 others were positive for *Giardia*. Pool records showed that no chlorine measurements had been taken on the day of the accidental faecal release and that no free chlorine level was detectable on the following day.

In 1988, an outbreak of giardiasis was associated with a hotel's new water slide pool (Greensmith et al., 1988). Among 107 hotel guests and visitors surveyed, 29 probable and 30 laboratory-confirmed cases of *Giardia* infection were found. Cases ranged from 3 to 58 years of age. Symptoms in the 59 cases included diarrhoea, cramps, foul-smelling stools, loss of appetite, fatigue, vomiting and weight loss. Significant associations were found between illness and staying at the hotel, using the water slide pool and swallowing pool water. A possible contributing factor was the proximity of a toddlers' pool, a potential source of faecal material, to the water slide pool. Water in the slide pool was treated by sand filtration and bromine disinfection.

2. Cryptosporidium-related outbreaks

A number of outbreaks of cryptosporidiosis have been linked to swimming pools. The sources of *Cryptosporidium* contaminating the pools were believed to be either sewage or the swimmers themselves. A number of outbreaks are reviewed below.

In 1988, an outbreak of 60 cases of cryptosporidiosis was reported in Los Angeles County, USA (CDC, 1990). Swimmers were exposed to pool water in which there had been a single accidental faecal release. The attack rate was about 73%. The common factor linking infected individuals was use of the swimming pool.

In August 1988, the first outbreak of cryptosporidiosis associated with a swimming pool in the United Kingdom was recognized following an increase in the number of cases of cryptosporidiosis that had been identified by the Doncaster Royal Infirmary microbiology laboratory (Joce et al., 1991). By October of that year, 67 cases had been reported. An investigation implicated one of two pools at a local sports centre. Oocysts were identified in the pool water. Inspection of the pool pipework revealed significant plumbing defects, which had allowed ingress of sewage from the main sewer into the circulating pool water. The epidemiological investigation confirmed an association between head immersion and illness. The concentration of oocysts detected in the pool water samples that were tested was 50 oocysts per litre. Difficulty had been experienced in controlling the level of free chlorine residual, which implied that disinfection was probably not maintained at an appropriate level.

An outbreak of cryptosporidiosis occurred in British Columbia, Canada, in 1990 (Bell et al., 1993). A case–control study and illness survey indicated that the transmission occurred in a public children's pool at the local recreation centre. Analysis using laboratory-confirmed cases showed that the illnesses were associated with swimming in the children's pool within two weeks before onset of illness. Attack rates ranged from 8% to 78% for various groups of children's pool users. Several accidental faecal releases, including diarrhoea, had occurred in the pool before and during the outbreak.

In 1992, public health officials in Oregon, USA, noted a large increase in the number of stool specimens submitted for parasitic examination that were positive for *Cryptosporidium* (McAnulty et al., 1994). They identified 55 patients with cryptosporidiosis, including 37 who were the first individuals ill in their households. A case–control study involving the first 18 case patients showed no association between illness and day-care attendance, drinking municipal drinking-water or drinking untreated surface waters. However, 9 of 18 case patients reported swimming at the local wave pool, whereas none of the controls indicated this activity. Seventeen case patients were finally identified as swimming in the same pool. The investigators concluded that the outbreak of cryptosporidiosis was probably caused by exposure to faecally contaminated pool water.

In August 1993, a parent informed the Department of Public Health of Madison, Wisconsin, USA, that her daughter was ill with a laboratory-confirmed *Cryptosporidium* infection and that members of her daughter's swim team had severe diarrhoea

(CDC, 1994). Fifty-five per cent of 31 pool users interviewed reported having had watery diarrhoea for two or more days. Forty-seven per cent of the 17 cases had had watery diarrhoea for more than five days. A second cluster of nine cases was identified later in the month. Seven of the nine reported swimming at a large outdoor pool. Public health authorities cleaned the pool, shock dosed with chlorine and prohibited people with diarrhoea from swimming in the pool.

In the UK, 18 outbreaks of cryptosporidiosis were associated with pools between 1989 and 1999. Recognized accidental faecal releases at the pool occurred in four of the outbreaks, although faecal contamination was known or suspected in a further five outbreaks. Outbreaks were associated with pools disinfected with chlorine and with ozone and with both well and poorly managed pools (PHLS, 2000).

Two protracted outbreaks of cryptosporidiosis associated with swimming pools were reported from Ohio and Nebraska, USA (CDC, 2001c). In both cases, accidental faecal releases (on more than one occasion) were observed. In the Nebraska outbreak, 32% of cases reported swimming during their illness or shortly afterwards.

In Australia, a statewide outbreak of cryptosporidiosis in New South Wales was associated with swimming at public pools (Puech et al., 2001). The association was reported to be stronger for cases from urban areas. The authors noted that *Cryptosporidium* oocysts were more commonly detected from pools where at least two notified cases had swum, and that outbreaks could involve multiple pools.

A large outbreak of cryptosporidiosis has been associated with a hotel in Majorca, Spain, used by British tourists. The outbreak was detected in Scotland, following the detection of cryptosporidiosis in tourists returning from Majorca. Almost 400 cases were identified, and the outbreak was thought to be associated with the hotel swimming pool, with oocysts being detected in samples of the pool water (Galmes et al., 2003). This outbreak resulted in guidelines on cryptosporidiosis prevention being produced for the Spanish hoteliers association (Confederación Española de Hoteles y Apartamentos Turísticos) and the UK Federation of Tour Operators (R. Cartwright, pers. comm.).

In the USA, an analysis of recreationally-associated waterborne outbreaks of illness between 2001 and 2002 was conducted (Yoder et al., 2004). *Cryptosporidium* species were the most common cause of gastrointestinal outbreaks of illness associated with treated swimming pool water.

3.3.3 Risk assessment

Giardia cysts are 4–12 μm in diameter. Viable cysts that are ingested by humans have an incubation period of about 7–12 days. The resulting gastroenteritis is characterized by diarrhoea with accompanying abdominal cramps. The illness lasts for about 7–10 days. *Cryptosporidium* oocysts are 4–6 μm in diameter and are much more resistant to chlorine than *Giardia* cysts. If viable oocysts are ingested, there is an incubation period of 4–9 days before symptoms appear. The illness lasts about 10–14 days, with symptoms typically including diarrhoea, vomiting and abdominal cramps. In patients with severely weakened immune systems, such as those with HIV infection and cancer and transplant patients taking certain immune system-suppressing drugs, cryptosporidiosis is generally chronic and more severe than in immunocompetent people and causes diarrhoea that can last long enough to be life threatening (Petersen, 1992).

The *Cryptosporidium* infective dose that affects 50% of the challenged population of humans is about 132 oocysts (DuPont et al., 1995), although this does depend upon the strain (Okhuysen et al., 1999), and for some strains fewer than 100 oocysts can lead to infection. The duration of shedding of these oocysts after infection is 1–2 weeks. The infection is self-limiting in most individuals, lasting 1–3 weeks. *Cryptosporidium* oocysts discharged by ill individuals are usually observed at densities of 10^6–10^7 per gram. The infective dose of *Giardia* that will cause gastroenteritis in 25% of an exposed population is 25 cysts. *Giardia* cysts discharged in the faeces of infected individuals are usually at densities of 3×10^6 per gram. The shedding of cysts can persist for up to six months (Table 3.5).

Table 3.5. Protozoan exposure factors

Agent	Density shed during infection[a]	Duration of shedding	Infective dose	Reference
Cryptosporidium	10^6–10^7 per gram	1–2 weeks	132/ID_{50}	Casemore, 1990; DuPont et al., 1995
Giardia	3×10^6 per gram	6 months	25/ID_{25}	Rendtorff, 1954; Feachem et al., 1983

ID_{50} (ID_{25}) – dose of microorganisms required to infect 50% (25%) of individuals exposed
[a] Figures represent the peak and are not representative of the whole of the infection period

3.3.4 Risk management

Giardia cysts and *Cryptosporidium* oocysts are very resistant to many disinfectants, including chlorine (Lykins et al., 1990). *Cryptosporidium*, for example (the more chlorine resistant of the two protozoa), requires chlorine concentrations of 30 mg/l for 240 min (at pH 7 and a temperature of 25 °C) for a 99% reduction to be achieved (i.e. an impractical level). Inactivation of oocysts with chlorine is greater when ozone, chlorine dioxide or UV irradiation is also used (Gregory, 2002). Ozone is a more effective disinfectant (compared with chlorine) for the inactivation of *Giardia* cysts and *Cryptosporidium* oocysts. *Cryptosporidium* oocysts are sensitive to 5 mg of ozone per litre. Almost all (99.9%) of the oocysts are killed after 1 min (at pH 7 and a temperature of 25 °C). Giardia cysts are sensitive to 0.6 mg of ozone per litre. Ninety per cent of the cysts are inactivated after 1 min (at pH 7 and a temperature of 5 °C). As ozone is not a residual disinfectant (i.e. it is not applied so as to persist in pool water in use), sufficient concentration and time for inactivation must be ensured during treatment before residual ozone removal and return to the pool.

It should be noted, however, that the figures above represent removal under laboratory (i.e. ideal) conditions. Additionally, studies have generally used oxidant demand-free water (i.e. they were not performed in simulated recreational water where additional organic material is present). Carpenter et al. (1999) found that the presence of faecal material increased the Ct value (disinfectant concentration in mg/l multiplied by time in minutes) needed to disinfect swimming pools.

UV is also effective at inactivating *Giardia* cysts and *Cryptosporidium* oocysts. A near complete inactivation (99.9%) of *Cryptosporidium* occurs at UV exposures of 10 mJ/cm²

(WHO, 2004). Inactivation of *Giardia* cysts (99%) occurs at lower UV intensities of 5 mJ/cm^2 (WHO, 2004). The efficacy of UV is impacted by particulate matter and the growth of biofilms. Thus, turbidity should be low, and UV lamps need to be cleaned periodically to remove biofilms or other substances that interfere with UV light emission. Like ozone, UV leaves no disinfectant residual and thus should be combined with chlorine or another disinfectant that remains in the water after treatment (WHO, 2004).

At present, the most practical approach to eliminating cysts and oocysts is through the use of filtration. *Cryptosporidium* oocysts are removed by filtration where the porosity of the filter is less than 4 μm. *Giardia* cysts are somewhat larger and are removed by filters with a porosity of 7 μm or less, although statistics on removal efficiency during filtration should be interpreted with caution. Removal and inactivation of cysts and oocysts occur only in the fraction of water passing through treatment. Since a pool is a mixed and not a plug flow system, the rate of reduction in concentration in the pool volume is slow.

Most outbreaks of giardiasis and cryptosporidiosis among pool swimmers have been linked to pools contaminated by sewage, accidental faecal releases or suspected accidental faecal releases. A study conducted in six pools in France, in the absence of detected faecal releases, found only a single instance when *Cryptosporidium* oocysts were detected (Fournier et al., 2002). An Italian investigation of 10 chlorinated swimming pools found *Cryptosporidium* and *Giardia* in 3% of pool water samples despite otherwise good water quality (according to microbial monitoring results) and free chlorine levels of approximately 1 mg/l. In addition, both *Cryptosporidium* and *Giardia* were always detected in the filter backwash water (Bonadonna et al., 2004). Pool maintenance and appropriate disinfection levels are easily overwhelmed by accidental faecal releases or sewage intrusion; therefore, the only possible response to this condition, once it has occurred, is to prevent use of the pool and physically remove the oocysts by draining or by applying a long period of filtration, as inactivation in the water volume (i.e. disinfection) is impossible (see Chapter 5). However, the best intervention is to prevent accidental faecal releases from occurring in the first place, through education of pool users about appropriate hygienic behaviour. Immunocompromised individuals should be aware that they are at increased risk of illness from exposure to pathogenic protozoa.

3.4 Non-faecally-derived bacteria

Infections and diseases associated with non-enteric pathogenic bacteria found in swimming pools and similar recreational water environments are summarized in Table 3.6. A number of these bacteria may be shed by bathers or may be present in biofilms (assemblages of surface-associated microbial cells enclosed in an extracellular matrix – Donlan, 2002). Biofilms may form on the lining of pipes (for example) in contact with water and may serve to protect the bacteria from disinfectants.

3.4.1 *Legionella* spp.

1. *Risk assessment*

Legionella are Gram-negative, non-spore-forming, motile, aerobic bacilli, which may be free-living or living within amoebae and other protozoa or within biofilms. *Legionella* spp. are heterotrophic bacteria found in a wide range of water environments and can proliferate at temperatures above 25 °C. They may be present in high numbers in natural spas using thermal spring water, and they can also grow in poorly main-

Table 3.6. Non-faecally-derived bacteria found in swimming pools and similar environments and their associated infections

Organism	Infection/disease	Source
Legionella spp.	Legionellosis (Pontiac fever and Legionnaires' disease)	Aerosols from natural spas, hot tubs and HVAC systems Poorly maintained showers or heated water systems
Pseudomonas aeruginosa	Folliculitis (hot tubs) Swimmer's ear (pools)	Bather shedding in pool and hot tub waters and on wet surfaces around pools and hot tubs
Mycobacterium spp.	Swimming pool granuloma Hypersensitivity pneumonitis	Bather shedding on wet surfaces around pools and hot tubs Aerosols from hot tubs and HVAC systems
Staphylococcus aureus	Skin, wound and ear infections	Bather shedding in pool water
Leptospira spp.	Haemorrhagic jaundice Aseptic meningitis	Pool water contaminated with urine from infected animals

HVAC – heating, ventilation and air conditioning

tained hot tubs, associated equipment and HVAC systems. *Legionella* spp. can also multiply on filter materials, namely granular activated carbon. However, exposure to *Legionella* is preventable through the implementation of basic management measures, including filtration, maintaining a continuous disinfectant residual in hot tubs (where disinfectants are not used, there must be a high dilution rate with fresh water) and the maintenance and physical cleaning of all natural spa, hot tub and pool equipment, including associated pipes and air-conditioning units.

The risk of infection following exposure to *Legionella* is difficult to assess and remains a matter of some debate (Atlas, 1999). Due to its prevalence in both natural and artificial environments, it must be considered that people are frequently exposed (at least to low numbers). Generally, there is no reaction to such exposure, asymptomatic production of antibodies or development of a mild flu-like illness, which may not be attributed to *Legionella* infection.

Legionella spp. can cause legionellosis, a range of pneumonic and non-pneumonic disease (WHO, 2005). Ninety per cent of cases of legionellosis are caused by *L. pneumophila*. Legionnaires' disease is characterized as a form of pneumonia. General risk factors for the illness include gender (males are roughly three times more likely than females to contract Legionnaires' disease), age (50 or older), chronic lung disease, cigarette smoking and excess consumption of alcohol. Specific risk factors, in relation to pools and hot tubs, include frequency of hot tub use and length of time spent in or around hot tubs. Although the attack rate is often less than 1%, mortality among hospitalized cases ranges widely up to 50%. Pontiac fever is a non-pneumonic, non-transmissible, non-fatal, influenza-like illness. The attack rate can be as high as 95% in the total exposed population. Patients with no underlying illness or condition recover in 2–5 days without treatment.

Risk of legionellosis from pools and similar environments is associated with proliferation of *Legionella* in spas or hot tubs, associated equipment and HVAC systems. The inference to be drawn from reported outbreaks and documented single cases is that inhalation of bacteria, or aspiration following ingestion, during natural spa or hot tub use may lead to disease, although Leoni et al. (2001) concluded that showers may present a greater risk of legionellosis than pool water. Thermal spring waters, especially, may be a source of high numbers of *Legionella* spp. (Bornstein et al., 1989; Martinelli et al., 2001), and they have been implicated in cases of legionnaires' disease (Bornstein et al., 1989; Mashiba et al., 1993).

Piped drinking-water distribution systems, household hot and cold water maintained between 25 °C and 50 °C, cooling towers, evaporative condensers of air-conditioning devices, water fountains and mist-generating machines are also potential sources of exposure to *Legionella*.

2. Risk management

Control of *Legionella* follows similar general principles to water safety plans applied to drinking-water supplies (WHO, 2004), although, in this instance, the principal responsibility will not lie with the water supplier. Authorities responsible for regulation of recreational facilities should ensure the implementation of safety plans, and such plans should address not only pools and hot tubs but also other water systems, including cooling towers and evaporative condensers operating at these facilities. As safety plans are limited to the recreational facility and the dose response is not easily described, adequate control measures should be defined in terms of practices that have been shown to be effective. Important control measures include appropriate design, to minimize the available surface area within the pool and hot tub system and associated pipework to reduce the area for possible bacterial colonization, ensuring an adequate disinfection residual in pools and hot tubs, proper maintenance and cleaning of equipment, and adequate ventilation.

Most of the reported legionellosis associated with recreational water use has been associated with hot tubs and natural spas (Groothuis et al., 1985; Althaus, 1986; Bornstein et al., 1989; Mashiba et al., 1993). Natural spa waters (especially thermal water) and associated equipment create an ideal habitat (warm, nutrient-containing aerobic water) for the selection and proliferation of *Legionella*. Hot tubs used for display in retail/wholesale outlets are also potential sources of infection (McEvoy et al., 2000). Outbreaks as a result of using swimming pools have not been reported (Marston et al., 1994), although *Legionella* spp. have been isolated from pool water and filter samples (Jeppesen et al., 2000; Leoni et al., 2001). Hot tubs integrated into larger swimming pool complexes appear to be less of a source of *Legionella* infection where shared water treatment facilities exist due to dilution of hot tub water into larger volumes of water for treatment.

Increased risk of *Legionella* in drinking-water has been associated with systems operating within the temperature range 25–50 °C. In hot tub facilities it is impractical to maintain a water temperature outside this range. Therefore, it is necessary to implement a range of other management strategies, which may include:

- ensuring a constant circulation of water in the hot tub;
- programming 'rest periods' during hot tub operation, in order to discourage excessive use and also to allow disinfectant levels to 'recover';
- frequent inspection and cleaning of all filters, including backwash filters (e.g. at least daily and when triggered by a pressure drop);

- cleaning pool surroundings, inspection of the physical conditions of the hot tub (e.g. daily);
- replacing at least half the water in each hot tub (e.g. daily);
- completely draining hot tubs and thoroughly cleaning all surfaces and all pipework (e.g. weekly);
- maintaining and physically cleaning heating, ventilation and air-conditioning systems serving the room in which hot tubs are located (e.g. weekly to monthly);
- inspection of the sand filter (e.g. quarterly); and
- ensuring staff are appropriately qualified and competent to operate the recreational facility.

In order to control the growth of *Legionella* in hot tubs and natural spas, physical cleaning of surfaces is critical, and high residual disinfectant concentrations may be required – e.g. free chlorine, where used, must be at least 1 mg/l at all times. Features such as water sprays, etc., in pool facilities should be periodically cleaned and flushed with a level of disinfectant adequate to eliminate *Legionella* spp. (e.g. by use of a solution of at least 5 mg of hypochlorite per litre).

Bathers should be encouraged to shower before entering the water. This will remove pollutants such as perspiration, cosmetics and organic debris that can act as a source of nutrients for bacterial growth and neutralize oxidizing biocides. Bather density and duration spent in hot tubs should also be controlled. Public and semi-public spa facilities should have programmed rest periods during the day. High-risk individuals (such as those with chronic lung disease) should be cautioned about the risks of exposure to *Legionella* in or around pools and hot tubs.

Operators of hot tub facilities should undertake a programme of verification of control measures, including:

- checking and adjusting residual disinfectant levels and pH (several times a day);
- inspection and maintenance of cleaning operations (daily to weekly); and
- where microbial testing for *Legionella* is undertaken, ensuring that *Legionella* levels are <1/100 ml.

3.4.2 *Pseudomonas aeruginosa*

1. *Risk assessment*

Pseudomonas aeruginosa is an aerobic, non-spore-forming, motile, Gram-negative, straight or slightly curved rod with dimensions 0.5–1 µm × 1.5–4 µm. It can metabolize a variety of organic compounds and is resistant to a wide range of antibiotics and disinfectants.

P. aeruginosa is ubiquitous in water, vegetation and soil. Although shedding from infected humans is the predominant source of *P. aeruginosa* in pools and hot tubs (Jacobson, 1985), the surrounding environment can be a source of contamination. The warm, moist environment on decks, drains, benches and floors provided by pools and similar environments is ideal for the growth of *Pseudomonas*, and it can grow well up to temperatures of 41 °C (Price & Ahearn, 1988). *Pseudomonas* tends to accumulate in biofilms in filters that are poorly maintained and in areas where pool hydraulics are poor (under moveable floors, for example). It is also likely that bathers pick up the organisms on their feet and hands and transfer them to the water. It has been proposed that the high water temperatures and turbulence in aerated hot tubs promote perspiration and desquamation (removal of skin cells). These materials protect organisms from exposure to disinfectants and contribute to the organic load, which, in turn, reduces the residual disinfectant level; they also act as a source of nutrients for the growth of *P. aeruginosa* (Kush & Hoadley, 1980; Ratnam et al., 1986; Price & Ahearn, 1988).

In one study, *P. aeruginosa* was isolated from all nine hot tubs examined (seven of which were commercial facilities and two domestic – Price & Ahearn, 1988). In the majority of hot tubs, concentrations ranged from 10^2 to 10^5 per ml. Locally recommended disinfection levels (of between 3 and 5 mg/l chlorine or bromine) were not maintained in any of the commercial hot tubs examined. In the same study, the two domestic hot tubs developed *P. aeruginosa* densities of 10^4–10^6 per ml within 24–48 h following stoppage of disinfection. In Northern Ireland, UK, Moore et al. (2002) found *P. aeruginosa* in 72% of hot tubs and 38% of swimming pools examined.

In hot tubs, the primary health effect associated with the presence of *P. aeruginosa* is folliculitis. Otitis externa and infections of the urinary tract, respiratory tract, wounds and cornea caused by *P. aeruginosa* have also been linked to hot tub use. Infection of hair follicles in the skin with *P. aeruginosa* produces a pustular rash, which may appear under surfaces covered with swimwear or may be more intense in these areas (Ratnam et al., 1986). The rash appears 48 h (range 8 h to 5 days) after exposure and usually resolves spontaneously within 5 days. It has been suggested that warm water supersaturates the epidermis, dilates dermal pores and facilitates their invasion by *P. aeruginosa* (Ratnam et al., 1986). There are some indications that extracellular enzymes produced by *P. aeruginosa* may damage skin and contribute to the bacteria's colonization (Highsmith et al., 1985). Other symptoms, such as headache, muscular aches, burning eyes and fever, have been reported. Some of these secondary symptoms resemble humidifier fever (Weissman & Schuyler, 1991) and therefore could be caused by the inhalation of *P. aeruginosa* endotoxins. Investigations have indicated that duration or frequency of exposure, bather loads, bather age and using the facility later in the day can be significant risk factors for folliculitis (Hudson et al., 1985; Ratnam et al., 1986; CDC, 2000). The sex of bathers does not appear to be a significant risk factor, but Hudson et al. (1985) suggest that women wearing one-piece bathing suits may be more susceptible to infection, presumably because one-piece suits trap more *P. aeruginosa*-contaminated water next to the skin. It has been suggested that the infective dose for healthy individuals is greater than 1000 organisms per ml (Price & Ahearn, 1988; Dadswell, 1997).

In swimming pools, the primary health effect associated with *P. aeruginosa* is otitis externa or swimmer's ear, although folliculitis has also been reported (Ratnam et al., 1986). Otitis externa is characterized by inflammation, swelling, redness and pain in the external auditory canal. Risk factors reported to increase the occurrence of otitis externa related to water exposure include amount of time spent in the water prior to the infection, less than 19 years of age and a history of previous ear infections (Seyfried & Cook, 1984; van Asperen et al., 1995). Repeated exposure to water is thought to remove the protective wax coating of the external ear canal, predisposing it to infection.

An indoor swimming pool with a system of water sprays has been implicated as the source of two sequential outbreaks of granulomatous pneumonitis among lifeguards (Rose et al., 1998). Inadequate chlorination led to the colonization of the spray circuits and pumps with Gram-negative bacteria, predominantly *P. aeruginosa*.

The bacteria and associated endotoxins were aerosolized and respired by the lifeguards when the sprays were activated. When the water spray circuits were replaced and supplied with an ozonation and chlorination system, there were no further occurrences of disease among personnel.

An outbreak of pseudomonas hot-foot syndrome, erythematous plantar nodules, has been reported as a result of exposure to a community wading pool. The floor of the pool was coated in abrasive grit, and the water contained high concentrations of *P. aeruginosa* (Fiorillo et al., 2001). Another outbreak occurred in Germany due to high concentrations of *P. aeruginosa* on the stairs to a water slide and resulted in some of the children being admitted to hospital (A. Wiedenmann, pers. comm.).

The true incidence of illnesses associated with *P. aeruginosa* in pools and similar environments is difficult to determine. Since the symptoms are primarily mild and self-limiting, most patients do not seek medical attention. In the USA, Yoder et al. (2004) reported 20 outbreaks of dermatitis between 2000 and 2001 associated with pools and hot tubs. In eight of these outbreaks *P. aeruginosa* was identified from water or filter samples; in the other 12 outbreaks *Pseudomonas* was suspected to be the cause. It was noted that contributing factors to these outbreaks included inadequate pool and hot tub maintenance and exceeding the bather load limit.

2. Risk management

Maintaining adequate residual disinfectant levels and routine cleaning are the key elements to controlling *P. aeruginosa* in swimming pools and similar recreational environments (see Chapter 5). While maintaining residual disinfectant levels in pools is relatively easy, the design and operation of some hot tubs make it difficult to achieve adequate disinfectant levels in these facilities. Under normal operating conditions, disinfectants can quickly dissipate (Highsmith et al., 1985; Price & Ahearn, 1988). In all facilities, frequent monitoring and adjustment of pH and disinfectant levels are essential. Most hot tubs use either chlorine- or bromine-based disinfectants. Shaw (1984) showed that chlorination was superior to bromine in controlling *P. aeruginosa*. He reported that during an outbreak investigation, *P. aeruginosa* could be isolated from water despite having a total bromine level of 5 mg/l and a pH of 7.5. Even in hot tubs with heterotrophic plate counts of <1 cfu/ml, *P. aeruginosa* was isolated from 5% of bromine-disinfected pools compared with only 0.8% of chlorine-disinfected pools (Shaw, 1984).

Routine, thorough cleaning of surrounding surfaces will help to reduce infections with *P. aeruginosa*. In addition, swimming pool, hot tub and natural spa operators should strongly encourage users to shower before entering the water and, where possible, control the number of bathers and their duration of hot tub exposure (Public Health Laboratory Service Spa Pools Working Group, 1994).

3.4.3 Mycobacterium spp.

1. Risk assessment

Mycobacterium spp. are rod-shaped bacteria that are 0.2–0.6 µm × 1.0–10 µm in size and have cell walls with a high lipid content. This feature means that they retain dyes in staining procedures that employ an acid wash; hence, they are often referred to as acid-fast bacteria. Atypical mycobacteria (i.e. other than strictly pathogenic species, such as *M. tuberculosis*) are ubiquitous in the aqueous environment and proliferate in and around swimming pools and similar environments (Leoni et al., 1999).

In pool environments, *M. marinum* is responsible for skin and soft tissue infections in normally healthy people. Infections frequently occur on abraded elbows and knees and result in localized lesions, often referred to as swimming pool granuloma. The organism is probably picked up from the pool edge by bathers as they climb in and out of the pool (Collins et al., 1984).

Respiratory illnesses associated with hot tub use in normally healthy individuals have been linked to other atypical mycobacteria (Embil et al., 1997; Kahana et al., 1997; Grimes et al., 2001; Khoor et al., 2001; Mangione et al., 2001; Cappelluti et al., 2003; Lumb et al., 2004). For example, *M. avium* in hot tub water has been linked to hypersensitivity pneumonitis and possibly pneumonia (Embil et al., 1997). Symptoms were flu-like and included cough, fever, chills, malaise and headaches. The illness followed the inhalation of heavily contaminated aerosols generated by the hot tub. The reported cases relate to domestic hot tubs, many of which were located outdoors. In most instances the frequency of hot tub use was high, as was the duration of exposure (an extreme example being use for 1–2 h each day), and maintenance of disinfection and cleaning were not ideal. It is likely that detected cases are only a small fraction of the total number of cases. Amoebae may also play a role in the transmission of *Mycobacterium* spp. (Cirillo et al., 1997).

2. Risk management

Mycobacteria are more resistant to disinfection than most bacteria due to the high lipid content of their cell wall (Engelbrecht et al., 1977). Therefore, thorough cleaning of surfaces and materials around pools and hot tubs where the organism may persist is necessary, supplemented by the maintenance of disinfection at appropriate levels. In addition, occasional shock dosing of chlorine (see Chapter 5) may be required to eradicate mycobacteria accumulated in biofilms within pool or hot tub components (Aubuchon et al., 1986). In natural spas where the use of disinfectants is undesirable or where it is difficult to maintain adequate disinfectant levels, superheating the water to 70 °C on a daily basis during periods of non-use may help to control *M. marinum* (Embil et al., 1997). Immunocompromised individuals should be cautioned about the risks of exposure to atypical mycobacteria in and around pools and hot tubs.

3.4.4 *Staphylococcus aureus*

1. Risk assessment

The genus *Staphylococcus* comprises non-motile, non-spore-forming and non-encapsulated Gram-positive cocci (0.5–1.5 μm in diameter) that ferment glucose and grow aerobically and anaerobically. They are usually catalase positive and occur singly and in pairs, tetrads, short chains and irregular grape-like clusters. In humans, there are three clinically important species – *Staphylococcus aureus*, *S. epidermidis* and *S. saprophyticus*. *S. aureus* is the only coagulase-positive species and is clinically the most important (Duerden et al., 1990).

Humans are the only known reservoir of *S. aureus*, and it is found on the anterior nasal mucosa and skin as well as in the faeces of a substantial portion of healthy individuals. Robinton & Mood (1966) found that *S. aureus* was shed by bathers under all conditions of swimming, and the bacteria can be found in surface films in pool water. Coagulase-positive *Staphylococcus* strains of normal human flora have been found in chlorinated swimming pools (Rocheleau et al., 1986).

The presence of *S. aureus* in swimming pools is believed to have resulted in skin rashes, wound infections, urinary tract infections, eye infections, otitis externa, impetigo and other infections (Calvert & Storey, 1988; Rivera & Adera, 1991). Infections of *S. aureus* acquired from recreational waters may not become apparent until 48 h after contact. De Araujo et al. (1990) have suggested that recreational waters with a high density of bathers present a risk of staphylococcal infection that is comparable to the risk of gastrointestinal illness involved in bathing in water considered unsafe because of faecal pollution. According to Favero et al. (1964) and Crone & Tee (1974), 50% or more of the total staphylococci isolated from swimming pool water samples are *S. aureus*. In Italy, however, in a study on chlorinated pools where the free chlorine level varied between 0.8 and 1.2 mg/l, *S. aureus* was not recovered from water samples (Bonadonna et al., 2004).

2. Risk management

Adequate inactivation of potentially pathogenic *S. aureus* in swimming pools can be attained by maintaining free chlorine levels greater than 1 mg/l (Keirn & Putnam, 1968; Rivera & Adera, 1991) or equivalent disinfection efficiency. There is evidence that showering before pool entry can reduce the shedding of staphylococci from the skin into the pool (Robinton & Mood, 1966). Continuous circulation of surface water through the treatment process helps to control the build-up of *S. aureus*. Pool contamination can also be reduced if the floors surrounding the pool and in the changing areas are kept at a high standard of cleanliness. Although it is not recommended that water samples be routinely monitored for *S. aureus*, where samples are taken, levels should be less than 100/100 ml.

3.4.5 *Leptospira interrogans sensu lato*

1. Risk assessment

Leptospires are motile spirochaete (helically coiled) bacteria. Traditionally, the genus *Leptospira* consists of two species, the pathogenic *L. interrogans* sensu lato and the saprophytic *L. biflexa* sensu lato. Serological tests within each species revealed many antigenic variations, and, on this basis, leptospires are classified as serovars. In addition, a classification system based on DNA relatedness is used (Brenner et al., 1999). The current species determination is based on this principle. The serological and genetic taxonomies are two different systems with only little correlation (Brenner et al., 1999). Free-living strains (*L. biflexa* sensu lato) are ubiquitous in the environment (Faine et al., 1999); the pathogenic strains (*L. interrogans* sensu lato), however, live in the kidneys of animal hosts.

Pathogenic leptospires live in the proximal renal tubules of the kidneys of carrier animals (including rats, cows and pigs) and are excreted in the urine, which can then contaminate surface waters. Humans and animals (humans are always incidental hosts) become infected either directly through contact with infected urine or indirectly via contact with contaminated water. Leptospires gain entry to the body through cuts and abrasions of the skin and through the mucosal surfaces of the mouth, nose and conjunctiva.

Diseases caused by *Leptospira interrogans* sensu lato have been given a variety of names, including swineherd's disease, Stuttgart disease and Weil's syndrome, but collectively all of these infections are termed leptospirosis. The clinical manifestations of leptospirosis vary considerably in form and intensity, ranging from a mild flu-like illness to a severe and potentially fatal form of the disease, characterized by liver and kidney failure and haemorrhages (Weil's syndrome). Severity is related to the infecting serovar as well as host characteristics, such as age and underlying health and nutritional status. Specific serovars are often associated with certain hosts.

Compared with many other pathogens, leptospires have a comparatively low resistance to adverse chemical and physical conditions, including disinfectants. They are seldom found in water of below pH 6.8, and they cannot tolerate drying or exposure to direct sunlight (Noguchi, 1918; Alston & Broom, 1958; Weyant et al., 1999).

The majority of reported outbreaks of waterborne leptospirosis have involved fresh recreational waters, but two outbreaks have been associated with non-chlorinated swimming pools (Cockburn et al., 1954; de Lima et al., 1990). Domestic or wild animals with access to the implicated waters were the probable sources of *Leptospira*.

2. Risk management

The risk of leptospirosis can be reduced by preventing direct animal access to swimming pools and maintaining adequate disinfectant concentrations. Informing users about the hazards of swimming in water that is accessible to domestic and wild animals may also help to prevent infections. Outbreaks are not common; thus, it appears that the risk of leptospirosis associated with swimming pools and hot tubs is low. Normal disinfection of pools is sufficient to inactivate *Leptospira* spp.

3.5 Non-faecally-derived viruses

Infections associated with non-faecally-derived viruses found in swimming pools and similar environments are summarized in Table 3.7.

Table 3.7. Non-faecally-derived viruses found in swimming pools and similar environments and their associated infections

Organism	Infection	Source
Adenoviruses[a]	Pharyngo-conjunctivitis (swimming pool conjunctivitis)	Other infected bathers
Molluscipoxvirus	Molluscum contagiosum	Bather shedding on benches, pool or hot tub decks, swimming aids
Papillomavirus	Plantar wart	Bather shedding on pool and hot tub decks and floors in showers and changing rooms

[a] Covered in Section 3.1.2

3.5.1 Molluscipoxvirus

1. Risk assessment

Molluscipoxvirus is a double-stranded DNA virus in the Poxviridae family. Virions are brick-shaped, about 320 nm × 250 nm × 200 nm. The virus causes molluscum contagiosum, an innocuous cutaneous disease limited to humans. It is spread by direct person-to-person contact or indirectly through physical contact with contaminated surfaces. The infection appears as small, round, firm papules or lesions, which grow to about 3–5 mm in diameter. The incubation period is 2–6 weeks or longer. Individual lesions persist for 2–4 months, and cases resolve spontaneously in 0.5–2 years. Swimming pool-related cases occur more frequently in children than in adults. The total number of annual cases is unknown. Since the infection is relatively innocuous, the reported number of cases is likely to be much less than the total number. Lesions are most often found on the arms, back of the legs and back, suggesting transmission through physical contact with the edge of the pool, benches around the pool, swimming aids carried into the pool or shared towels (Castilla et al., 1995). Indirect transmission via water in swimming pools is not likely. Although cases associated with hot tubs have not been reported, they should not be ruled out as a route of exposure.

2. Risk management

The only source of molluscipoxvirus in swimming pool and similar facilities is infected bathers (Oren & Wende, 1991). Hence, the most important means of controlling the spread of the infection is to educate the public about the disease, the importance of limiting contact between infected and non-infected people and medical treatment. Thorough frequent cleaning of surfaces in facilities that are prone to contamination can reduce the spread of the disease.

3.5.2 Papillomavirus

1. Risk assessment

Papillomavirus is a double-stranded DNA virus in the family Papovaviridae. The virions are spherical and approximately 55 nm in diameter. The virus causes benign cutaneous tumours in humans. An infection that occurs on the sole (or plantar surface) of the foot is referred to as a verruca plantaris or plantar wart. Papillomaviruses are extremely resistant to desiccation and thus can remain infectious for many years. The incubation period of the virus remains unknown, but it is estimated to be 1–20 weeks. The infection is extremely common among children and young adults between the ages of 12 and 16 who frequent public pools and hot tubs. It is less common among adults, suggesting that they acquire immunity to the infection. At facilities such as public swimming pools, plantar warts are usually acquired via direct physical contact with shower and changing room floors contaminated with infected skin fragments (Conklin, 1990; Johnson, 1995). Papillomavirus is not transmitted via pool or hot tub waters.

2. Risk management

The primary source of papillomavirus in swimming pool facilities is infected bathers. Hence, the most important means of controlling the spread of the virus is to educate the public about the disease, the importance of limiting contact between infected and non-infected people and medical treatment. The use of pre-swim showering, wearing of sandals in showers and changing rooms and regular cleaning of surfaces in swimming pool facilities that are prone to contamination can reduce the spread of the virus.

3.6 Non-faecally-derived protozoa

Table 3.8 summarizes the non-faecally-derived protozoa found in or associated with swimming pools and similar environments and their associated infections.

Table 3.8. Non-faecally-derived protozoa found in swimming pools and similar environments and their associated infections

Organism	Infection	Source
Naegleria fowleri	Primary amoebic meningoencephalitis (PAM)	Pools, hot tubs and natural spas including water and components
Acanthamoeba spp.	Acanthamoeba keratitis Granulomatous amoebic encephalitis (GAE)	Aerosols from HVAC systems
Plasmodium spp.	Malaria	Seasonally used pools may provide a breeding habitat for mosquitoes carrying *Plasmodium*

HVAC – heating, ventilation and air conditioning

3.6.1 *Naegleria fowleri*

1. Risk assessment

Naegleria fowleri is a free-living amoeba (i.e. it does not require the infection of a host organism to complete its life cycle) present in fresh water and soil. The life cycle includes an environmentally resistant encysted form. Cysts are spherical, 8–12 μm in diameter, with smooth, single-layered walls containing one or two mucus-plugged pores through which the trophozoites (infectious stages) emerge. *N. fowleri* is thermophilic, preferring warm water and reproducing successfully at temperatures up to 46 °C.

N. fowleri causes primary amoebic meningoencephalitis (PAM). Infection is usually acquired by exposure to water in ponds, natural spas and artificial lakes (Martinez & Visvesvara, 1997; Szenasi et al., 1998). Victims are usually healthy children and young adults who have had contact with water about 7–10 days before the onset of symptoms (Visvesvara, 1999). Infection occurs when water containing the organisms is forcefully inhaled or splashed onto the olfactory epithelium, usually from diving, jumping or underwater swimming. The amoebae in the water then make their way into the brain and central nervous system. Symptoms of the infection include severe headache, high fever, stiff neck, nausea, vomiting, seizures and hallucinations. The infection is not contagious. For those infected, death occurs usually 3–10 days after onset of symptoms. Respiratory symptoms occur in some patients and may be the result of hypersensitivity or allergic reactions or may represent a subclinical infection (Martinez & Visvesvara, 1997).

Although PAM is an extremely rare disease, cases have been associated with pools and natural spas. In Usti, Czech Republic, 16 cases of PAM were associated with a public swimming pool (Cerva & Novak, 1968). The source of the contamination was traced to a cavity behind a false wall used to shorten the pool length. The pool took water from a local river, which was the likely source of the organism. One confirmed case of PAM occurred in Bath Spa, in the UK, in 1978. The victim was a young girl who swam in a public swimming pool fed with water from the historic thermal springs that rise naturally in the city (Cain et al., 1981). Subsequent analysis confirmed the thermal springs to be the source of the infection (Kilvington et al., 1991). *N. fowleri* has also been isolated from air-conditioning units (Martinez, 1993).

2. *Risk management*

Risk of infection can be reduced by minimizing the occurrence of the causative agent through appropriate choice of source water, proper cleaning, maintenance, coagulation–filtration and disinfection.

3.6.2 *Acanthamoeba spp.*

1. *Risk assessment*

Several species of free-living *Acanthamoeba* are human pathogens (*A. castellanii, A. culbertsoni, A. polyphaga*). They can be found in all aquatic environments, including disinfected swimming pools. Under adverse conditions, they form a dormant encysted stage. Cysts measure 15–28 μm, depending on the species. *Acanthamoeba* cysts are highly resistant to extremes of temperature, disinfection and desiccation. The cysts will retain viability from –20 °C to 56 °C. When favourable conditions occur, such as a ready supply of bacteria and a suitable temperature, the cysts hatch (excyst) and the trophozoites emerge to feed and replicate. All pathogenic species will grow at 36–37 °C, with an optimum of about 30 °C. Although *Acanthamoeba* is common in most environments, human contact with the organism rarely leads to infection.

Human pathogenic species of *Acanthamoeba* cause two clinically distinct diseases: granulomatous amoebic encephalitis (GAE) and inflammation of the cornea (keratitis) (Ma et al., 1990; Martinez, 1991; Kilvington & White, 1994).

GAE is a chronic disease of the immunosuppressed; GAE is either subacute or chronic but is invariably fatal. Symptoms include fever, headaches, seizures, meningitis and visual abnormalities. GAE is extremely rare, with only 60 cases reported worldwide. The route of infection in GAE is unclear, although invasion of the brain may result from the blood following a primary infection elsewhere in the body, possibly the skin or lungs (Martinez, 1985, 1991). The precise source of such infections is unknown because of the almost ubiquitous presence of *Acanthamoeba* in the environment.

Acanthamoeba keratitis affects previously healthy people and is a severe and potentially blinding infection of the cornea (Ma et al., 1990; Kilvington & White, 1994). In the untreated state, acanthamoeba keratitis can lead to permanent blindness. Although only one eye is usually affected, cases of bilateral infection have been reported. The disease is characterized by intense pain and ring-shaped infiltrates in the corneal stroma. Contact lens wearers are most at risk from the infection and account for approximately 90% of reported cases (Kilvington & White, 1994). Poor contact lens hygiene practices (notably ignoring recommended cleaning and disinfection procedures and rinsing or storing of lenses in tap water or non-sterile saline solutions) are recognized risk factors, although the wearing of contact lenses while swimming or participating in other water sports may also be a risk factor. In non-contact lens related keratitis, infection arises from trauma to the eye and contamination with environmental matter such as soil and water (Sharma et al., 1990). Samples et al. (1984) report a case of keratitis that may have been acquired from domestic hot tub use.

2. *Risk management*

Although *Acanthamoeba* cysts are resistant to chlorine- and bromine-based disinfectants, they can be removed by filtration. Thus, it is unlikely that properly operated swimming pools and similar environments would contain sufficient numbers of cysts to cause infection in normally healthy individuals. Immunosuppressed individuals who use swimming pools, natural spas or hot tubs should be aware of the increased risk of GAE. A number of precautionary measures are available to contact lens wearers, including removal before entering the water, wearing goggles, post-swim contact lens wash using appropriate lens fluid and use of daily disposable lenses.

3.6.3 *Plasmodium spp.*

1. Risk assessment

Swimming pools are associated not with *Plasmodium* spp. but with anopheline mosquito larvae, the insect vectors of *Plasmodium*. Mbogo et al. (submitted) found that over 70% of swimming pools sampled in urban Malindi in Kenya were positive for mosquito larvae. The problem relates to the seasonal use of the pools. Before people leave their summer houses, it is common to drain the pool; however, rainwater accumulated during the rainy season provides a suitable habitat for mosquito breeding, with the attendant risks of malaria as a result.

2. Risk management

During the rains, when the pools fill with water, they should be drained every 5–7 days to avoid mosquito larvae developing into adults. The swimming pools may also be treated with appropriate larvicides when not in use for long periods.

3.7 Non-faecally-derived fungi

Infections associated with fungi found in swimming pools and similar environments are summarized in Table 3.9.

Table 3.9. Fungi found in swimming pools and similar environments and their associated infections

Organism	Infection	Source
Trichophyton spp. *Epidermophyton floccosum*	Athlete's foot (tinea pedis)	Bather shedding on floors in changing rooms, showers and pool or hot tub decks

3.7.1 *Trichophyton spp. and Epidermophyton floccosum*

1. Risk assessment

Epidermophyton floccosum and various species of fungi in the genus *Trichophyton* cause superficial fungal infections of the hair, fingernails or skin. Infection of the skin of the foot (usually between the toes) is described as tinea pedis or, more commonly, as 'athlete's foot' (Aho & Hirn, 1981). Symptoms include maceration, cracking and scaling of the skin, with intense itching. Tinea pedis may be transmitted by direct person-to-person contact; in swimming pools, however, it may be transmitted by physical contact with surfaces, such as floors in public showers, changing rooms, etc., contaminated with infected skin fragments. In Japan, a study comparing students attending a regular swimming class with those who did not found a significantly greater level of infection in the swimmers (odds ratio of 8.5), and *Trichophyton* spp. were isolated from the floor of a hot tub and the floor of one of the changing rooms (Kamihama et al., 1997). The fungus colonizes the stratum corneum when environmental conditions, particularly humidity, are optimal. From in vitro experiments, it has been calculated that it takes approximately 3–4 h for the fungus to initiate infection. The infection is common among lifeguards and competitive swimmers, but relatively benign; thus, the true number of cases is unknown.

2. Risk management

The sole source of these fungi in swimming pool and similar facilities is infected bathers. Hence, the most important means of controlling the spread of the fungus is to educate the public about the disease, the importance of limiting contact between infected and non-infected bathers and medical treatment. The use of pre-swim showers, wearing of sandals in showers and changing rooms and frequent cleaning of surfaces in swimming pool facilities that are prone to contamination can reduce the spread of the fungi (Al-Doory & Ramsey, 1987). People with severe athlete's foot or similar dermal infections should not frequent public swimming pools, natural spas or hot tubs. Routine disinfection appears to control the spread of these fungi in swimming pools and similar environments (Public Health Laboratory Service Spa Pools Working Group, 1994).

3.8 References

Aho R, Hirn H (1981) A survey of fungi and some indicator bacteria in chlorinated water of indoor public swimming pools. *Zentralblatt für Bakteriologie, Mikrobiologie und Hygiene B*, 173: 242–249.

Al-Doory Y, Ramsey S (1987) Cutaneous mycotic diseases. In: *Moulds and health: Who is at risk?* Springfield, IL, Charles C. Thomas, pp. 61–68, 206–208.

Alston JM, Broom JC (1958) *Leptospirosis in man and animals*. Edinburgh, Livingstone Ltd.

Althaus H (1986) Legionellas in swimming pools. *A.B. Archiv des Badewesens*, 38: 242–245.

Atlas RM (1999) *Legionella*: from environmental habitats to disease pathology, detection and control. *Environmental Microbiology*, 1(4): 283–293.

Aubuchon C, Hill JJ, Graham DR (1986) Atypical mycobacterial infection of soft tissue associated with use of a hot tub. *Journal of Bone and Joint Surgery*, 68-A(5): 766–/768.

Bell A, Guasparini R, Meeds D, Mathias RG, Farley JD (1993) A swimming pool associated outbreak of cryptosporidiosis in British Columbia. *Canadian Journal of Public Health*, 84: 334–337.

Blostein J (1991) Shigellosis from swimming in a park in Michigan. *Public Health Reports*, 106: 317–322.

Bonadonna L, Briancesco R, Magini V, Orsini M, Romano-Spica V (2004) [A preliminary investigation on the occurrence of protozoa in swimming pools in Italy.] *Annali di Igiene Medicina Preventiva e di Comunità*, 16(6): 709–720 (in Italian).

Bornstein N, Marmet D, Surgot M, Nowicki M, Arslan A, Esteve J, Fleurette J (1989) Exposure to Legionellaceae at a hot spring spa: a prospective clinical and serological study. *Epidemiology and Infection*, 102: 31–36.

Brenner DJ, Kaufmann AF, Sulzer KR, Steigerwalt AG, Rogers FC, Weyant RS (1999) Further determination of DNA relatedness between serogroups and serovars in the family Leptospiraceae with a proposal for *Leptospira alexanderi* sp. Nov and four new *Leptospira* genomospecies. *International Journal of Systematic Bacteriology*, 49: 833–858.

Brewster DH, Brown MI, Robertson D, Houghton GL, Bimson J, Sharp JCM (1994) An outbreak of *Escherichia coli* O157 associated with a children's paddling pool. *Epidemiology and Infection*, 112: 441–447.

Cain ARR, Wiley PF, Brownell B, Warhurst DC (1981) Primary amoebic meningoencephalitis. *Archives of Diseases in Childhood*, 56: 140–143.

Caldwell GG, Lindsey NJ, Wulff H, Donnelly DD, Bohl FN (1974) Epidemic with adenovirus type 7 acute conjunctivitis in swimmers. *American Journal of Epidemiology*, 99: 230–234.

Calvert J, Storey A (1988) Microorganisms in swimming pools – are you looking for the right one? *Journal of the Institution of Environmental Health Officers*, 96(7): 12.

Cappelluti E, Fraire AE, Schaefer OP (2003) A case of 'hot tub lung' due to *Mycobacterium avium* complex in an immunocompetent host. *Archives of Internal Medicine*, 163: 845–848.

Carpenter C, Fayer R, Trout J, Beach MJ (1999) Chlorine disinfection of recreational water for *Cryptosporidium parvum*. *Emerging Infectious Diseases*, 5(4): 579–584.

Casemore DP (1990) Epidemiological aspects of human cryptosporidiosis. *Epidemiology and Infection*, 104: 1–28.

Castilla MT, Sanzo JM, Fuentes S (1995) Molluscum contagiosum in children and its relationship to attendance at swimming-pools: an epidemiological study. *Dermatology*, 191(2): 165.

CDC (1990) Swimming-associated cryptosporidiosis – Los Angeles County. *Morbidity and Mortality Weekly Report*, 39: 343–345.

CDC (1994) *Cryptosporidium* infections associated with swimming pools – Dane County, Wisconsin. *Morbidity and Mortality Weekly Report*, 43: 561–563.

CDC (1996) Lake-associated outbreak of *Escherichia coli* O157-H7 – Illinois. *Morbidity and Mortality Weekly Report*, 45: 437–439.

CDC (2000) *Pseudomonas* dermatitis/folliculitis associated with pools and hot tubs – Colorado and Maine, 1999–2000. *Morbidity and Mortality Weekly Report*, 49: 1087–1091.

CDC (2001a) Prevalence of parasites in fecal material from chlorinated swimming pools – United States, 1999. *Morbidity and Mortality Weekly Report*, 50: 410–412.

CDC (2001b) Shigellosis outbreak associated with an unchlorinated fill-and-drain wading pool – Iowa, 2001. *Morbidity and Mortality Weekly Report*, 50(37): 797–800.

CDC (2001c) Protracted outbreaks of cryptosporidiosis associated with swimming pool use – Ohio and Nebraska, 2000. *Morbidity and Mortality Weekly Report*, 50(20): 406–410.

CDC (2004) An outbreak of norovirus gastroenteritis at a swimming club – Vermont, 2004. *Morbidity and Mortality Weekly Report*, 53: 793–795.

CDSC (1995) Surveillance of waterborne diseases. *Communicable Disease Report Weekly*, 5: 129.

CDSC (1997) Surveillance of waterborne disease and water quality: January to June 1997. *Communicable Disease Report Weekly*, 7: 317–319.

CDSC (1998) Surveillance of waterborne disease and water quality: January to June 1998. *Communicable Disease Report Weekly*, 8: 305–306.

CDSC (1999) Surveillance of waterborne disease and water quality: January to June 1999, and summary of 1998. *Communicable Disease Report Weekly*, 9: 305–308.

CDSC (2000) Surveillance of waterborne disease and water quality: July to December 1999. *Communicable Disease Report Weekly*, 10: 65–68.

Cerva L, Novak K (1968) Amoebic meningoencephalitis: sixteen fatalities. *Science*, 160: 92.

Cirillo JD, Falkow S, Tompkins LS, Bermudez LE (1997) Interaction of *Mycobacterium avium* with environmental amoebae enhances virulence. *Infection and Immunity*, 65(9): 3759–3767.

Cockburn TA, Vavra JD, Spencer SS, Dann JR, Peterson LJ, Reinhard KR (1954) Human leptospirosis associated with a swimming pool diagnosed after eleven years. *American Journal of Hygiene*, 60: 1–7.

Collins CH, Grange JM, Yates MD (1984) A review. *Mycobacterium* in water. *Journal of Applied Bacteriology*, 57(2): 193–211.

Conklin RJ (1990) Common cutaneous disorders in athletes. *Sports Medicine*, 9: 100–119.

Coulepis AG, Locarnini SA, Lehmann NI, Gust ID (1980) Detection of hepatitis A virus in the feces of patients with naturally acquired infections. *Journal of Infectious Diseases*, 141(2): 151–156.

Cransberg K, van den Kerkhof JH, Banffer JR, Stijnen C, Wernors K, van de Kar NC, Nauta J, Wolff ED (1996) Four cases of hemolytic uremic syndrome – source contaminated swimming water? *Clinical Nephrology*, 46: 45–49.

Crone PB, Tee GH (1974) Staphylococci in swimming pool water. *Journal of Hygiene (London)*, 73(2): 213–220.

D'Angelo LJ, Hierholzer JC, Keenlyside RA, Anderson LJ, Martone WJ (1979) Pharyngo-conjunctival fever caused by adenovirus type 4: Recovery of virus from pool water. *Journal of Infectious Diseases*, 140: 42–47.

Dadswell J (1997) Poor swimming pool management: how real is the health risk? *Environmental Health*, 105(3): 69–73.

de Araujo MA, Guimaraes VF, Mendonca-Hagler LCS, Hagler AN (1990) *Staphylococcus aureus* and faecal streptococci in fresh and marine waters of Rio de Janeiro, Brazil. *Revista de Microbiologia*, 21(2): 141–147.

de Lima SC, Sakata EE, Santo CE, Yasuda PH, Stiliano SV, Ribeiro FA (1990) Outbreak of human leptospirosis by recreational activity in the municipality of Sao Jose dos Campos, Sao Paulo. Seroepidemiological study. *Revista do Instituto de Medicina Tropical de Sao Paulo*, 32(6): 474–479.

Donlan R (2002) Biofilms: microbial life on surfaces. *Emerging Infectious Diseases*, 8(9): 881–890.

Duerden BI, Reid TMS, Jewsbury JM, Turk DC (1990) *Microbial and parasitic infection*. London, Edward Arnold, pp. 74–76.

DuPont HL (1988) *Shigella. Infectious Disease Clinics of North America*, 2(3): 599–605.

DuPont HL, Chappell CL, Sterling CR, Okhuysen PC, Rose JB, Jakubowski W (1995) The infectivity of *Cryptosporidium parvum* in healthy volunteers. *New England Journal of Medicine*, 332(13): 855–859.

Embil J, Warren P, Yakrus M, Corne S, Forrest D, Hershfield E (1997) Pulmonary illness associated with exposure to *Mycobacterium-avium* complex in hot tub water. *Chest*, 111(3): 534–536.

Engelbrecht RS, Severnin BF, Massarik MT, Faroo S, Lee SH, Haas CN, Lalchandani A (1977) *New microbial indicators of disinfection efficiency*. Washington, DC, United States Environmental Protection Agency (Report No. EPA 600/2-77-052).

Faine S, Adler B, Bolin C, Perolat P (1999) *Leptospira and leptospirosis*, 2nd ed. Melbourne, MediSci, 272 pp.

Favero MS, Drake CH, Randall GB (1964) Use of staphylococci as indicators of swimming pool pollution. *Public Health Reports*, 79: 61–70.

Feachem RG, Bradley DJ, Garelick H, Mara DD (1983) *Sanitation and disease: Health aspects of excreta and wastewater management*. New York, NY, John Wiley and Sons.

Fiorillo L, Zucker M, Sawyer D, Lin AN (2001) The pseudomonas hot-foot syndrome. *New England Journal of Medicine*, 345(5): 335–338.

Fournier S, Dubrou S, Liguory O, Gaussin F, Santillana-Hayat M, Sarfati C, Molina JM, Derouin F (2002) Detection of microsporidia, cryptosporidia and giardia in swimming pools: a one-year prospective study. *FEMS Immunology and Medical Microbiology*, 33: 209–213.

Fox JP, Brandt CD, Wassermann FE, Hall CE, Spigland CE, Kogan A, Elveback LR (1969) The Virus Watch Program: A continuing surveillance of viral infections in metropolitan New York families. VI. Observations of adenovirus infections; virus excretion patterns, antibody response, efficiency of surveillance patterns of infection and relation to illness. *American Journal of Epidemiology*, 89: 25–50.

Foy HM, Cooney MK, Hatlen JB (1968) Adenovirus type 3 epidemic associated with intermittent chlorination of a swimming pool. *Archives of Environmental Health*, 17: 795–802.

Galmes A, Nicolau A, Arbona G, Gomis E, Guma M, Smith-Palmer A, Hernandez-Pezzi G, Soler P (2003) Cryptosporidiosis outbreak in British tourists who stayed at a hotel in Majorca, Spain. *Eurosurveillance Weekly*, 7(33).

Gray SF, Gunnell DJ, Peters TJ (1994) Risk factors for giardiasis: a case–control study in Avon and Somerset. *Epidemiology and Infection*, 113: 95–102.

Greensmith CT, Stanwick RS, Elliot BE, Fast MV (1988) Giardiasis associated with the use of a water slide. *Pediatric Infectious Diseases Journal*, 7: 91–94.

Gregory R (2002) Bench-marking pool water treatment for coping with *Cryptosporidium*. *Journal of Environmental Health Research*, 1: 11–18.

Grimes MM, Cole TJ, Fowler III AA (2001) Obstructive granulomatous bronchiolitis due to *Mycobacterium avium* complex in an immunocompetent man. *Respiration*, 68: 411–415.

Groothuis DG, Havelaar AH, Veenendaal HR (1985) A note on legionellas in whirlpools. *Journal of Applied Bacteriology*, 58(5): 479–481.

Harley D, Harrower B, Lyon M, Dick A (2001) A primary school outbreak of pharyngoconjunctival fever caused by adenovirus type 3. *Communicable Diseases Intelligence*, 25(1): 9–12.

Harter L, Frost F, Grunenfelder G, Perkins-Jones K, Libby J (1984) Giardiasis in an infant and toddler swim class. *American Journal of Public Health*, 74: 155–156.

Highsmith AK, Le PN, Khabbaz RF, Munn VP (1985) Characteristics of *Pseudomonas aeruginosa* isolated from whirlpools and bathers. *Infection Control*, 6(10): 407–412.

Hildebrand JM, Maguire HC, Halliman RE, Kangesu E (1996) An outbreak of *Escherichia* coli O157 infection linked to paddling pools. *Communicable Disease Report Review*, 6: R33–R36.

Hudson PJ, Vogt RL, Jillson DA, Kappel SJ, Highsmith AK (1985) Duration of whirlpool-spa use as a risk factor for *Pseudomonas* dermatitis. *American Journal of Epidemiology*, 122: 915–917.

Hunt DA, Sebugwawo S, Edmondson SG, Casemore DP (1994) Cryptosporidiosis associated with a swimming pool complex. *Communicable Disease Report Review*, 4(2): R20–R22.

Hunter PR (1997) Adenoviral infections. *Waterborne disease: Epidemiology and ecology*. Chichester, John Wiley & Sons.

Jacobson JA (1985) Pool-associated *Pseudomonas aeruginosa* dermatitis and other bathing-associated infections. *Infection Control*, 6: 398–401.

Jeppesen C, Bagge L, Jeppesen VF (2000) [*Legionella pneumophila* in pool water.] *Ugeskrift for Laeger*, 162: 3592–3594 (in Danish).

Joce RE, Bruce J, Kiely D, Noah ND, Dempster WB, Stalker R, Gumsley P, Chapman PA, Norman P, Watkins J, Smith HV, Price TJ, Watts D (1991) An outbreak of cryptosporidiosis associated with a swimming pool. *Epidemiology and Infection*, 107: 497–508.

Johnson LW (1995) Communal showers and the risk of plantar warts. *Journal of Family Practice*, 40: 136–138.

Kahana LM, Kay JM, Yakrus MA, Waserman S (1997) *Mycobacterium avium* complex infection in an immunocompetent young adult related to hot tub exposure. *Chest*, 111: 242–245.

Kamihama T, Kimura T, Hosokawa J-I, Ueji M, Takase T, Tagami K (1997) Tinea pedis outbreak in swimming pools in Japan. *Public Health*, 111: 249–253.

Kappus KD, Marks JS, Holman RC, Bryant JK, Baker C, Gary GW, Greenberg HB (1982) An outbreak of Norwalk gastroenteritis associated with swimming in a pool and secondary person to person transmission. *American Journal of Epidemiology*, 116: 834–839.

Kee F, McElroy G, Stewart D, Coyle P, Watson J (1994) A community outbreak of echovirus infection associated with an outdoor swimming pool. *Journal of Public Health Medicine*, 16: 145–148.

Keene WE, McAnulty JM, Hoesly FC, Williams LP Jr, Hedberg K, Oxman GL, Barrett TJ, Pfaller MA, Fleming DW (1994) A swimming-associated outbreak of hemorrhagic colitis caused by *Escherichia coli* O157:H7 and *Shigella sonnei*. *New England Journal of Medicine*, 331(9): 579–584.

Keirn MA, Putnam HD (1968) Resistance of staphylococci to halogens as related to a swimming pool environment. *Health Laboratory Science*, 5(3): 180–193.

Khoor A, Leslie KO, Tazelaar HD, Helmers RA, Colby TV (2001) Diffuse pulmonary disease caused by nontuberculous mycobacteria in immunocompetent people (hot tub lung). *American Journal of Clinical Pathology*, 115: 755–762.

Kidd AH, Jonsson M, Garwicz D, Kajon AE, Wermenbol AG, Verweij XX, de Jong JC (1996) Rapid sub-genus identification of human adenovirus isolates. *Journal of Clinical Microbiology*, 34: 622–627.

Kilvington S, White DG (1994) *Acanthamoeba*: biology, ecology and human disease. *Reviews in Medical Microbiology*, 5: 12–20.

Kilvington S, Mann PG, Warhurst DC (1991) Pathogenic *Naegleria* amoebae in the waters of Bath: a fatality and its consequences. In: Kellaway GA, ed. *Hot springs of Bath*. Bath, Bath City Council, pp. 89–96.

Kush BJ, Hoadley AW (1980) A preliminary survey of the association of *Ps. aeruginosa* with commercial whirlpool bath waters. *American Journal of Public Health*, 70: 279–281.

Leoni E, Legnani P, Mucci MT, Pirani R (1999) Prevalence of mycobacteria in a swimming pool environment. *Journal of Applied Microbiology*, 87: 683–688.

Leoni E, Legnani PP, Bucci Sabattini MA, Righi F (2001) Prevalence of *Legionella* spp. in swimming pool environment. *Water Research*, 35(15): 3749–3753.

Lumb R, Stapledon R, Scroop A, Bond P, Cunliffe D, Goodwin A, Doyle R, Bastian I (2004) Investigation of spa pools associated with lung disorders caused by *Mycobacterium avium* complex in immunocompetent adults. *Applied and Environmental Microbiology*, 70(8): 4906–4910.

Lykins BW, Goodrich JA, Hoff JC (1990) Concerns with using chlorine-dioxide disinfection in the U.S.A. *Journal of Water Supply: Research and Technology – AQUA*, 39: 376–386.

Ma P, Visvesvara GS, Martinez AJ, Theodore FH, Dagget PM, Sawyer TK (1990) *Naegleria* and *Acanthamoeba* infections: review. *Reviews of Infectious Diseases*, 12: 490–513.

Mahoney FJ, Farley TA, Kelso KY, Wilson SA, Horan JM, McFarland LM (1992) An outbreak of hepatitis A associated with swimming in a public pool. *Journal of Infectious Diseases*, 165: 613–618.

Makintubee S, Mallonee J, Istre GR (1987) Shigellosis outbreak associated with swimming. *American Journal of Public Health*, 77: 166–168.

Mangione EJ, Huitt G, Lenaway D, Beebe J, Baily A, Figoski M, Rau MP, Albrecht KD, Yakrus MA (2001) Nontuberculous mycobacterial disease following hot tub exposure. *Emerging Infectious Diseases*, 7: 1039–1042.

Marston BJ, Lipman HB, Breiman RF (1994) Surveillance for Legionnaires' disease: Risk factors for morbidity and mortality. *Archives of Internal Medicine*, 154(21): 2417–2422.

Martinelli F, Carasi S, Scarcella C, Speziani F (2001) Detection of *Legionella pneumophila* at thermal spas. *New Microbiology*, 24: 259–264.

Martinez AJ (1985) *Free-living amebas: natural history, prevention, diagnosis, pathology, and treatment of disease*. Boca Raton, FL, CRC Press.

Martinez AJ (1991) Infections of the central nervous system due to *Acanthamoeba*. *Reviews of Infectious Diseases*, 13: S399–S402.

Martinez AJ (1993) Free-living amebas: infection of the central nervous system. *Mount Sinai Journal of Medicine*, 60(4): 271–278.

Martinez AJ, Visvesvara GS (1997) Free-living, amphizoic and opportunistic amebas. *Brain Pathology*, 7(1): 583–598.

Martone WJ, Hierholzer JC, Keenlyside RA, Fraser DW, D'Angelo LJ, Winkler WG (1980) An outbreak of adenovirus type 3 disease at a private recreation center swimming pool. *American Journal of Epidemiology*, 111: 229–237.

Mashiba K, Hamamoto T, Torikai K (1993) [A case of Legionnaires' disease due to aspiration of hot spring water and isolation of *Legionella pneumophila* from hot spring water.] *Kansenshogaku Zasshi*, 67: 163–166 (in Japanese).

Maunula L, Kalso S, von Bonsdorff C-H, Pönkä A (2004) Wading pool water contaminated with both noroviruses and astroviruses as the source of a gastroenteritis outbreak. *Epidemiology and Infection*, 132: 737–743.

Mbogo CM, Kahindi S, Githeko AK, Keating J, Kibe L, Githure JI, Beier JC (submitted) Ecology of malaria vectors and culicine abundance in urban Malindi, Kenya. *Journal of Vector Ecology*.

McAnulty JM, Fleming DW, Gonzalez AH (1994) A community-wide outbreak of cryptosporidiosis associated with swimming at a wave pool. *Journal of the American Medical Association*, 272: 1597–1600.

McEvoy M, Batchelor N, Hamilton G, MacDonald A, Faiers M, Sills A, Lee J, Harrison T (2000) A cluster of cases of legionnaires' disease associated with exposure to a spa pool on display. *Communicable Disease and Public Health*, 3(1):43–45.

Moore JE, Heaney N, Millar BC, Crowe M, Elborn JS (2002) Incidence of *Pseudomonas aeruginosa* in recreational and hydrotherapy pools. *Communicable Disease and Public Health*, 5(1): 23–26.

Noguchi H (1918) The survival of *Leptospira* (*Spirochaeta*) *icterohaemorrhagie* in nature: observations concerning micro-chemical reactions and intermediate hosts. *Journal of Experimental Medicine*, 17: 609–614.

Okhuysen PC, Chappell CL, Crabb JH, Sterling CR, DuPont HL (1999) Virulence of three distinct *Cryptosporidium parvum* isolates for healthy adults. *Journal of Infectious Diseases*, 180: 1275–1281.

Oren B, Wende SO (1991) An outbreak of molluscum contagiosum in a kibbutz. *Infection*, 19: 159–161.

Pai CH, Gordon R, Sims HB, Bryon LE (1984) Sporadic cases of hemorrhagic colitis associated with *Escherichia* coli O157:H7. *Annals of Internal Medicine*, 101: 738–742.

Papapetropoulou M, Vantarakis AC (1998) Detection of adenovirus outbreak at a municipal swimming pool by nested PCR amplification. *Journal of Infection*, 36: 101–103.

Petersen C (1992) Cryptosporidiosis in patients with the human immunodeficiency virus. *Clinical Infectious Diseases*, 15: 903–909.

PHLS (2000) *Review of outbreaks of cryptosporidiosis in swimming pools*. Marlow, Foundation for Water Research, Public Health Laboratory Service (DWI0812).

Porter JD, Ragazzoni HP, Buchanon JD, Waskin HA, Juranek DD, Parkin WE (1988) *Giardia* transmission in a swimming pool. *American Journal of Public Health*, 78(6): 659–662.

Price D, Ahearn DG (1988) Incidence and persistence of *Pseudomonas aeruginosa* in whirlpools. *Journal of Clinical Microbiology*, 26: 1650–1654.

Public Health Laboratory Service Spa Pools Working Group (1994) *Hygiene for spa pools*. London, Blackmore Press (ISBN 0 901144 371).

Puech MC, McAnulty JM, Lesjak M, Shaw N, Heron L, Watson JM (2001) A statewide outbreak of cryptosporidiosis in New South Wales associated with swimming at public pools. *Epidemiology and Infection*, 126: 389–396.

Ratnam S, Hogan K, March SB, Butler RW (1986) Whirlpool-associated folliculitis caused by *Pseudomonas aeruginosa*: Report of an outbreak and review. *Journal of Clinical Microbiology*, 23(3): 655–659.

Rendtorff RC (1954) The experimental transmission of human intestinal protozoan parasites. II. *Giardia lamblia* cysts given in capsules. *American Journal of Hygiene*, 59: 209–220.

Rivera JB, Adera T (1991) Assessing water quality. Staphylococci as microbial indicators in swimming pools. *Journal of Environmental Health*, 53(6): 29–32.

Robinton ED, Mood EW (1966) A quantitative and qualitative appraisal of microbial pollution of water by swimmers: a preliminary report. *Journal of Hygiene (London)*, 64(4): 489–499.

Rocheleau S, Desjardins R, Lafrance P, Briere F (1986) Control of bacteria populations in public pools. *Sciences et Techniques de l'eau*, 19: 117–128.

Rose CS, Martyny JW, Newman LS, Milton DK, King TE Jr, Beebe JL, McCammon JB, Hoffman RE, Kreiss K (1998) "Lifeguard lung": Endemic granulomatous pneumonitis in an indoor swimming pool. *American Journal of Public Health*, 88(12): 1795–1800.

Samples JR, Binder PS, Luibel FJ, Font RL, Visvesvara GS, Peter CR (1984) Acanthamoeba keratitis possibly acquired from a hot tub. *Archives of Ophthalmology*, 102: 707–710.

SCA (1995) *Methods for the examination of waters and associated materials*. Standing Committee of Analysts. London, HMSO.

Seyfried PL, Cook RJ (1984) Otitis externa infections related to *Pseudomonas aeruginosa* levels in five Ontario lakes. *Canadian Journal of Public Health*, 75: 83–90.

Sharma S, Srinivasan M, George C (1990) *Acanthamoeba* keratitis in non-contact lens wearers. *Archives of Ophthalmology*, 108: 676–678.

Shaw JH (1984) A retrospective comparison of the effectiveness of bromination and chlorination in controlling *Pseudomonas aeruginosa* in spas (whirlpools) in Alberta. *Canadian Journal of Public Health*, 75: 61–68.

Solt K, Nagy T, Csohan A, Csanady M, Hollos I (1994) [An outbreak of hepatitis A due to a thermal spa.] *Budapesti Kozegeszsegugy*, 26(1): 8–12 (in Hungarian).

Sorvillo FJ, Waterman SH, Vogt JK, England B (1988) Shigellosis associated with recreational water contact in Los Angeles County. *American Journal of Tropical Medicine and Hygiene*, 38(3): 613–617.

Sundkist T, Dryden M, Gabb R, Soltanpoor N, Casemore D, Stuart J (1997) Outbreak of cryptosporidiosis associated with a swimming pool in Andover. *Communicable Disease Report Review*, 7: R190–R192.

Szenasi Z, Endo T, Yagita K, Nagy E (1998) Isolation, identification and increasing importance of 'free-living' amoebae causing human disease. *Journal of Medical Microbiology*, 47(1): 5–16.

Turner M, Istre GR, Beauchamp H, Baum M, Arnold S (1987) Community outbreak of adenovirus type 7a infections associated with a swimming pool. *Southern Medical Journal*, 80: 712–715.

van Asperen IA, de Rover CM, Schijven JF, Oetomo SB, Schellekens JF, van Leeuwen NJ, Colle C, Havelaar AH, Kromhout D, Sprenger MW (1995) Risk of otitis externa after swimming in recreational fresh water lakes containing *Pseudomonas aeruginosa*. *British Medical Journal*, 311: 1407–1410.

Visvesvara GS (1999) Pathogenic and opportunistic free-living amebae. In: Murray PR, Baron EJ, Pfaller MA, Tenover FC, Yolken RH, eds. *Manual of clinical microbiology*, 7th ed. Washington, DC, ASM Press, pp. 1383–1384.

Weissman DN, Schuyler MR (1991) Biological agents and allergenic diseases. In: Samet JM, Spengler JD, eds. *Indoor air pollution: a health perspective*. Baltimore, MD, Johns Hopkins University Press.

Weyant RS, Bragg SL, Kaufmann AF (1999) *Leptospira* and leptonema. In: Murray PR, Baron EJ, Pfaller MA, Tenover FC, Yolken RH, eds. *Manual of clinical microbiology*, 7th ed. Washington, DC, ASM Press.

WHO (2004) *Guidelines for drinking-water quality*, 3rd ed., *Vol. 1: Recommendations*. Geneva, World Health Organization.

WHO (2005) *Legionella and the prevention of legionellosis*. Geneva, World Health Organization, in preparation.

Wyn-Jones AP, Sellwood J (2001) Enteric viruses in the aquatic environment. *Journal of Applied Microbiology*, 91: 945–962.

Yoder JS, Blackburn BG, Craun GF, Hill V, Levy DA, Chen N, Lee SH, Calderon RL, Beach MJ (2004) Surveillance of waterborne-disease outbreaks associated with recreational water – United States, 2001–2002. *Morbidity and Mortality Weekly Report Surveillance Summaries*, 53: 1–22.

CHAPTER 4
Chemical hazards

Chemicals found in pool water can be derived from a number of sources: the source water, deliberate additions such as disinfectants and the pool users themselves (see Figure 4.1). This chapter describes the routes of exposure to swimming pool chemicals, the chemicals typically found in pool water and their possible health effects.

While there is clearly a need to ensure proper consideration of health and safety issues for operators and pool users in relation to the use and storage of swimming pool chemicals, this aspect is not covered in this volume.

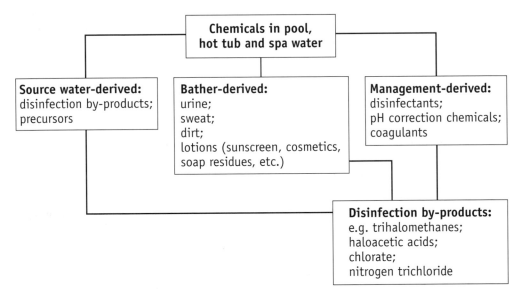

Figure 4.1. Possible pool water contaminants in swimming pools and similar environments

4.1 Exposure

There are three main routes of exposure to chemicals in swimming pools and similar environments:

- direct ingestion of water;
- inhalation of volatile or aerosolized solutes; and
- dermal contact and absorption through the skin.

4.1.1 Ingestion

The amount of water ingested by swimmers and pool users will depend upon a range of factors, including experience, age, skill and type of activity. The duration of exposure will vary significantly in different circumstances, but for adults, extended exposure would be expected to be associated with greater skill (e.g. competitive swimmers), and so there would be a lower rate of ingestion in a comparable time than for less skilled users. The situation with children is much less clear. There appear to be no data with which to make a more detailed assessment. A number of estimates have been made of possible intakes while participating in activities in swimming pools and similar environments, with the most convincing being a pilot study by Evans et al. (2001). This used urine sample analysis, with 24-h urine samples taken from swimmers who had used a pool disinfected with dichloroisocyanurate and analysed for cyanurate concentrations. All the participants swam, but there is no information on the participant swimming duration. This study found that the average water intake by children (37 ml) was higher than the intake by adults (16 ml). In addition, the intake by adult men (22 ml) was higher than that by women (12 ml); the intake by boys (45 ml) was higher than the intake by girls (30 ml). The upper 95th percentile intake was for children and was approximately 90 ml. This was a small study, but the data are of high quality compared with most other estimates, and the estimates, are based upon empirical data rather than assumptions. In this volume, a 'worst case' intake of 100 ml for a child is assumed in calculating ingestion exposure to chemicals in pool water.

4.1.2 Inhalation

Swimmers and pool users inhale from the atmosphere just above the water's surface, and the volume of air inhaled is a function of the intensity of effort and time. Individuals using an indoor pool also breathe air in the wider area of the building housing the pool. However, the concentration of pool-derived chemical in the pool environment will be considerably diluted in open air pools. Inhalation exposure will be largely associated with volatile substances that are lost from the water surface, but will also include some inhalation of aerosols, within a hot tub (for example) or where there is significant splashing. The normal assumption is that an adult will inhale approximately 10 m^3 of air during an 8-h working day (WHO, 1999). However, this will also depend on the physical effort involved. There will, therefore, be significant individual variation depending upon the type of activity and level of effort.

4.1.3 Dermal contact

The skin will be extensively exposed to chemicals in pool water. Some may have a direct impact on the skin, eyes and mucous membranes, but chemicals present in pool water may also cross the skin of the pool, hot tub or spa user and be absorbed into the body. Two pathways have been suggested for transport across the stratum corneum (outermost layer of skin): one for lipophilic chemicals and the other for hydrophilic chemicals (Raykar et al., 1988). The extent of uptake through the skin will depend on a range of factors, including the period of contact with the water, the temperature of the water and the concentration of the chemical.

4.2 Source water-derived chemicals

All source waters contain chemicals, some of which may be important with respect to pool, hot tub and spa safety. Water from a municipal drinking-water supply may contain organic materials (such as humic acid, which is a precursor of disinfection by-products), disinfection by-products (see Section 4.5) from previous treatment/disinfection processes, lime and alkalis, phosphates and, for chloraminated systems, monochloramines. Seawater contains high bromide concentrations. In some circumstances, radon may also be present in water that is derived from groundwater. Under such circumstances, adequate ventilation in indoor pools and hot tubs will be an important consideration. WHO is considering radon in relation to drinking-water quality guidelines and other guidance.

4.3 Bather-derived chemicals

Nitrogen compounds, particularly ammonia, that are excreted by bathers (in a number of ways) react with free disinfectant to produce several by-products. A number of nitrogen compounds can be eluted from the skin (Table 4.1). The nitrogen content in sweat is around 1 g/l, primarily in the form of urea, ammonia, amino acids and creatinine. Depending on the circumstances, the composition of sweat varies widely. Significant amounts of nitrogen compounds can also be discharged into pool water via urine (Table 4.1). The urine release into swimming pools has been variously estimated to average between 25 and 30 ml per bather (Gunkel & Jessen, 1988) and be as high as 77.5 ml per bather (Erdinger et al., 1997a), although this area has not been well researched.

The distribution of total nitrogen in urine among relevant nitrogen compounds (Table 4.1) has been calculated from statistically determined means of values based on 24-h urine samples. Although more than 80% of the total nitrogen content in urine is present in the form of urea and the ammonia content (at approximately 5%) is low, swimming pool water exhibits considerable concentrations of ammonia-derived compounds in the form of combined chlorine and nitrate. It therefore appears that there is degradation of urea following chemical reactions with chlorine.

Table 4.1. Nitrogen-containing compounds in sweat and urine[a]

Nitrogen-containing compounds	Sweat		Urine	
	Mean content (mg/l)	Portion of total nitrogen (%)	Mean content (mg/l)	Portion of total nitrogen (%)
Urea	680	68	10 240	84
Ammonia	180	18	560	5
Amino acids	45	5	280	2
Creatinine	7	1	640	5
Other compounds	80	8	500	4
Total nitrogen	992	100	12 220	100

[a] Adapted from Jandik, 1977

In a study on the fate of chlorine and organic materials in swimming pools using analogues of body fluids and soiling in a model pool, the results showed that organic carbon, chloramines and trihalomethanes all reached a steady state after 200–500 h of operation. Only insignificant amounts of the volatile by-products were found to be lost to the atmosphere, and only nitrate was found to accumulate, accounting for 4–28% of the dosed amino nitrogen (Judd & Bullock, 2003). No information is available on concentrations of chemicals in actual swimming pool water from cosmetics, suntan oil, soap residues, etc.

4.4 Management-derived chemicals

A number of management-derived chemicals are added to pool water in order to achieve the required water quality. A proportion of pool water is constantly undergoing treatment, which generally includes filtration (often in conjunction with coagulation), pH correction and disinfection (see Chapter 5).

4.4.1 Disinfectants

A range of disinfectants are used in swimming pools and similar environments. The most common are outlined in Table 4.2 (and covered in more detail in Chapter 5). They are added in order to inactivate pathogens and other nuisance microorganisms. Chlorine, in one of its various forms, is the most widely used disinfectant.

Some disinfectants, such as ozone and UV, kill or inactivate microorganisms as the water undergoes treatment, but there is no lasting disinfectant effect or 'residual' that reaches the pool and continues to act upon chemicals and microorganisms in the water. Thus, where these types of disinfection are used, a chlorine- or bromine-type disinfectant is also employed to provide continued disinfection. The active available disinfectant in the water is referred to as 'residual' or, in the case of chlorine, 'free' to distinguish it from combined chlorine (which is not a disinfectant). In the case of

Table 4.2. Disinfectants and disinfecting systems used in swimming pools and similar environments

Disinfectants used most frequently in large, heavily used pools	Disinfectants used in smaller pools and hot tubs	Disinfectants used for small-scale and domestic pools
Chlorine • Gas • Calcium/sodium hypochlorite • Electrolytic generation of sodium hypochlorite • Chlorinated isocyanurates (generally outdoor pools) Bromochlorodimethylhydantoin (BCDMH) Chlorine dioxide[a] Ozone[a] UV[a]	Bromine • Liquid bromine • Sodium bromide + hypochlorite Lithium hypochlorite	Bromide/hypochlorite UV[a] UV–ozone[a] Iodine Hydrogen peroxide/ silver/copper Biguanide

[a] Usually used in combination with residual disinfectants (i.e. chlorine- or bromine-based)

bromine, as the combined form is also a disinfectant, there is no need to distinguish between the two, so 'total' bromine is measured.

The type and form of disinfectant need to be chosen with respect to the specific requirements of the pool. In the case of small and domestic pools, important requirements are easy handling and ease of use as well as effectiveness. In all cases, the choice of disinfectant must be made after consideration of the efficacy of a disinfectant under the circumstances of use (more details are given in Chapter 5) and the ability to monitor disinfectant levels.

1. *Chlorine-based disinfectants*

Chlorination is the most widely used pool water disinfection method, usually in the form of chlorine gas, sodium, calcium or lithium hypochlorite but also with chlorinated isocyanurates. These are all loosely referred to as 'chlorine'.

Practice varies widely around the world, as do the levels of free chlorine that are currently considered to be acceptable in order to achieve adequate disinfection while minimizing user discomfort. For example, free chlorine levels of less than 1 mg/l are considered acceptable in some countries, while in other countries allowable levels may be considerably higher. Due to the nature of hot tubs (warmer water, often accompanied by aeration and a greater user to water volume ratio), acceptable free chlorine levels tend to be higher than in swimming pools. It is recommended that acceptable levels of free chlorine continue to be set at the local level, but in public and semi-public pools these should not exceed 3 mg/l and in public/semi-public hot tubs these should not exceed 5 mg/l. Lower free chlorine concentrations may be health protective when combined with other good management practices (e.g. pre-swim showering, effective coagulation and filtration, etc.) or when ozone or UV is also used.

Using high levels of chlorine (up to 20 mg/l) as a shock dose (see Chapter 5) as a preventive measure or to correct specific problems may be part of a strategy of proper pool management. While it should not be used to compensate for inadequacies of other management practices, periodic shock dosing can be an effective tool to maintain microbial quality of water and to minimize build-up of biofilms and chloramines (see Sections 4.5 and 5.3.4).

Chlorine in solution at the concentrations recommended is considered to be toxicologically acceptable even for drinking-water; the WHO health-based guideline value for chlorine in drinking-water is 5 mg/l (WHO, 2004). Concentrations significantly in excess of this may not be of health significance with regard to ingestion (as no adverse effect level was identified in the study used), even though there might be some problems regarding eye and mucous membrane irritation. The primary issues would then become acceptability to swimmers.

The chlorinated isocyanurates are stabilized chlorine compounds, which are widely used in the disinfection of outdoor or lightly loaded swimming pools. They dissociate in water to release free chlorine in equilibrium with cyanuric acid. A residual of cyanuric acid and a number of chlorine/cyanuric acid products will be present in the water. The Joint FAO/WHO Expert Committee on Food Additives and Contaminants (JECFA) has considered the chlorinated isocyanurates with regard to drinking-water disinfection and proposed a tolerable daily intake (TDI) for anhydrous sodium dichloroisocyanurate (NaDCC) of 0–2 mg/kg of body weight (JECFA, 2004). This would translate into an intake of 20 mg of NaDCC per day (or 11.7 mg of cyanuric acid per day) for a 10-kg child. To avoid consuming the TDI, assuming 100 ml of pool water is swallowed in a session would mean that the concentration of cyanuric acid/chlorinated isocyanurates should be kept below 117 mg/l. Levels of cyanuric acid should be kept between 50 and 100 mg/l in order not to interfere with the release of free chlorine, and it is recommended that levels should not exceed 100 mg/l. However, although no comprehensive surveys are available, there are a number of reported measurements of high levels of cyanuric acid in pools and hot tubs in the USA. Sandel (1990) found an average concentration of 75.9 mg/l with a median of 57.5 mg/l and a maximum of 406 mg/l. Other studies have reported that 25% of pools (122 of 486) had cyanuric acid concentrations greater than 100 mg/l (Rakestraw, 1994) and as high as 140 mg/l (Latta, 1995). Unpublished data from the Olin Corporation suggest that levels up to 500 mg/l may be found. Regular dilution with fresh water (see Chapter 5) is required in order to keep cyanuric acid at an acceptable concentration.

2. Chlorine dioxide

Chlorine dioxide is not classed as a chlorine-based disinfectant, as it acts in a different way and does not produce free chlorine. Chlorine dioxide breaks down to chlorite and chlorate, which will remain in solution; the WHO health-based drinking-water provisional guideline value for chlorite is 0.7 mg/l (based on a TDI of 0.03 mg/kg of body weight) (WHO, 2004), and this is also the provisional guideline for chlorate. There is potential for a build-up of chlorite/chlorate in recirculating pool water with time. In order to remain within the TDI levels of chlorate and chlorite, they should be maintained below 3 mg/l (assuming a 10-kg child and an intake of 100 ml).

3. Bromine-based disinfectants

Liquid bromine is not commonly used in pool disinfection. Bromine-based disinfectants for pools are available in two forms, bromochlorodimethylhydantoin (BCDMH) and a two-part system that consists of sodium bromide and an oxidizer (usually hypochlorite). As with chlorine-based disinfectants, local practice varies, and acceptable total bromine may be as high as 10 mg/l. Although there is limited evidence about bromine toxicity, it is recommended that total bromine does not exceed 2.0–2.5 mg/l. The use of bromine-based disinfectants is generally not practical for outdoor pools and spas because the bromine residual is depleted rapidly in sunlight (MDHSS, undated).

There are reports that a number of swimmers in brominated pools develop eye and skin irritation (Rycroft & Penny, 1983). However, Kelsall & Sim (2001) in a study examining three different pool disinfection systems (chlorine, chlorine/ozone and bromine/ozone) did not find that the bromine disinfection system was associated with a greater risk of skin rashes, although the number of bathers studied was small.

4. Ozone and ultraviolet

Ozone and UV radiation purify the pool water as it passes through the plant room, and neither leaves residual disinfectant in the water. They are, therefore, used in conjunction with conventional chlorine- and bromine-based disinfectants. The primary health issue in ozone use in swimming pool disinfection is the leakage of ozone into the atmosphere from ozone generators and contact tanks, which need to be properly ventilated to the outside atmosphere. It is also appropriate to include a deozonation step in the treatment process, to prevent carry-over in the treated water. Ozone is a severe respiratory irritant, and it is, therefore, important that ozone concentrations in the atmosphere of the pool building are controlled. The air quality guideline value of 0.12 mg/m³ (WHO, 2000) is an appropriate concentration to protect bathers and staff working in the pool building.

5. *Other disinfectants*

Other disinfectant systems may be used, especially in small pools. Hydrogen peroxide used with silver and copper ions will normally provide low levels of the silver and copper ions in the water. However, it is most important that proper consideration is given to replacement of water to prevent excessive build-up of the ions. A similar situation would apply to biguanide, which is also used as a disinfectant in outdoor pools.

4.4.2 pH correction

The chemical required for pH value adjustment will generally depend on whether the disinfectant used is itself alkaline or acidic. Alkaline disinfectants (e.g. sodium hypochlorite) normally require only the addition of an acid for pH correction, usually a solution of sodium hydrogen sulfate, carbon dioxide or hydrochloric acid. Acidic disinfectants (e.g. chlorine gas) normally require the addition of an alkali, usually a solution of sodium carbonate (soda ash). There should be no adverse health effects associated with the use of these chemicals provided that they are dosed correctly and the pH range is maintained between 7.2 and 8.0 (see Section 5.10.3).

4.4.3 Coagulants

Coagulants (e.g. polyaluminium chloride) may be used to enhance the removal of dissolved, colloidal or suspended material. These work by bringing the material out of solution or suspension as solids and then clumping the solids together to produce a floc. The floc is then trapped during filtration.

4.5 Disinfection by-products (DBP)

Disinfectants can react with other chemicals in the water to give rise to by-products (Table 4.3). Most information available relates to the reactions of chlorine, as will be seen from Tables 4.4–4.11. Although there is potentially a large number of chlorine-derived disinfection by-products, the substances produced in the greatest quantities are the trihalomethanes (THMs), of which chloroform is generally present in the greatest concentration, and the haloacetic acids (HAAs), of which di- and trichloroacetic acid are generally present in the greatest concentrations (WHO, 2000). It is probable that a range of organic chloramines could be formed, depending on the nature of the precursors and pool conditions. Data on their occurrence in swimming pool waters are relatively limited, although they are important in terms of atmospheric contamination in enclosed pools and hot tubs.

When inorganic bromide is present in the water, this can be oxidized to form bromine, which will also take part in the reaction to produce brominated by-products such as the brominated THMs. This means that the bromide/hypochlorite system of disinfection would be expected to give much higher proportions of the brominated by-products. Seawater pools disinfected with chlorine would also be expected to show a high proportion of brominated by-products since seawater contains significant levels of bromide. Seawater pools might also be expected to show a proportion of iodinated by-products in view of the presence of iodide in the water. In all pools in which free halogen (i.e. chlorine, bromine or iodine) is the primary disinfectant, no matter what form the halogen donor takes, there will be a range of by-products, but these will be

Table 4.3. Predominant chemical disinfectants used in pool water treatment and their associated disinfection by-products[a]

Disinfectant	Disinfection by-products
Chlorine/hypochlorite	trihalomethanes
	haloacetic acids
	haloacetonitriles
	haloketones
	chloral hydrate (trichloroacetaldehyde)
	chloropicrin (trichloronitromethane)
	cyanogen chloride
	chlorate
	chloramines
Ozone	bromate
	aldehydes
	ketones
	ketoacids
	carboxylic acids
	bromoform
	brominated acetic acids
Chlorine dioxide	chlorite
	chlorate
Bromine/hypochlorite	trihalomethanes, mainly bromoform
BCDMH	bromal hydrate
	bromate
	bromamines

[a] UV is a physical system and is generally not considered to produce by-products

found at significantly lower concentrations than the THMs and HAAs. The use of ozone in the presence of bromide can lead to the formation of bromate, which can build up over time without adequate dilution with fresh water (see Chapter 5).

While chlorination has been relatively well studied, it must be emphasized that data on ozonation by-products and other disinfectants are very limited. Although those by-products found commonly in ozonated drinking-water would be expected, there appear to be few data on the concentrations found in swimming pools and similar environments.

Both chlorine and bromine will react, extremely rapidly, with ammonia in the water, to form chloramines (monochloramine, dichloramine and nitrogen trichloride) and bromamines (collectively known as haloamines). The mean content of urea and ammonia in urine is 10 240 mg/l and 560 mg/l, respectively (Table 4.1), but hydrolysis of urea will give rise to more ammonia in the water (Jandik, 1977). Nitrogen-containing organic compounds, such as amino acids, may react with hypochlorite to form organic chloramines (Taras, 1953; Isaak & Morris, 1980).

During storage, chlorate can build up within sodium hypochlorite solution, and this can contribute to chlorate levels in disinfected water. However, it is unlikely to be of concern to health unless the concentrations are allowed to reach excessive levels (i.e. >3 mg/l), in which case the efficacy of the hypochlorite is likely to be compromised.

Ozone can react with residual bromide to produce bromate, which is quite stable and can build up over time (Grguric et al., 1994). This is of concern in drinking-water systems but will be of lower concern in swimming pools. However, if ozone were used to disinfect seawater pools, the concentration of bromate would be expected to be potentially much higher. In addition, bromate is a by-product of the electrolytic generation of hypochlorite if the brine used is high in bromide. Ozone also reacts with organic matter to produce a range of oxygenated substances, including aldehydes and carboxylic acids. Where bromide is present, it can also result in the formation of brominated products similar to liquid bromine.

More data are required on the impact of UV on disinfection by-products when used in conjunction with residual disinfectants. UV disinfection is not considered to produce by-products, and it seems to significantly reduce the levels of chloramines.

4.5.1 *Exposure to disinfection by-products*

While swimming pools have not been studied to the same extent as drinking-water, there are some data on the occurrence and concentrations of a number of disinfection by-products in pool water, although the data are limited to a small number of the major substances. A summary of the concentrations of various prominent organic by-products of chlorination (THMs, HAAs, haloacetonitriles and others) measured in different pools is provided in Table 4.4 and Tables 4.9–4.11 below. Many of these data are relatively old and may reflect past management practices. Concentrations will vary as a consequence of the concentration of precursor compounds, disinfectant dose, residual disinfectant level, temperature and pH. The THM found in the greatest concentrations in freshwater pools is chloroform, while in seawater pools, it is usually bromoform (Baudisch et al., 1997; Gundermann et al., 1997).

1. *Trihalomethanes*

Sandel (1990) examined data from 114 residential pools in the USA and reported average concentrations of chloroform of 67.1 µg/l with a maximum value of 313 µg/l. In hot spring pools, the median concentration of chloroform was 3.8 µg/l and the maximum was 6.4 µg/l (Erdinger et al., 1997b). Fantuzzi et al. (2001) reported total THM concentrations of 17.8–70.8 µg/l in swimming pools in Italy. In a study of eight swimming pools in London, Chu & Nieuwenhuijsen (2002) collected and analysed pool water samples for total organic carbon (TOC) and THMs. They reported a geometric mean[1] for all swimming pools of 5.8 mg/l for TOC, 125.2 µg/l for total THMs and 113.3 µg/l for chloroform; there was a linear correlation between the number of people in the pool and the concentration of THMs. The pool concentrations of disinfection by-products will also be influenced by the concentration of THMs and the potential precursor compounds in the source and make-up water.

THMs are volatile in nature and can be lost from the surface of the water, so they will also be found in the air above indoor pools (Table 4.5). Transport from swimming pool water to the air will depend on a number of factors, including the concentration in the pool water, the temperature and the amount of splashing and surface

---

[1] Mean values in Table 4.4 are arithmetic means.

disturbance. The concentrations at different levels in the air above the pool will also depend on factors such as ventilation, the size of the building and the air circulation. Fantuzzi et al. (2001) examined THM levels in five indoor pools in Italy and found mean concentrations of total THMs in poolside air of 58.0 $\mu g/m^3 \pm 22.1$ $\mu g/m^3$ and concentrations of 26.1 $\mu g/m^3 \pm 24.3$ $\mu g/m^3$ in the reception area.

Strähle et al. (2000) studied the THM concentrations in the blood of swimmers compared with the concentrations of THMs in pool water and ambient air (Table 4.6). They showed that intake via inhalation was probably the major route of uptake of volatile components, since the concentration of THMs in the outdoor pool water was higher than the concentration in the indoor pool water, but the concentrations in air above the pool and in blood were higher in the indoor pool than in the outdoor pool. This would imply that good ventilation at pool level would be a significant contributor to minimizing exposure to THMs. Erdinger et al. (2004) found that in a study in which subjects swam with and without scuba tanks, THMs were mainly taken up by the respiratory pathway and only about one third of the total burden was taken up through the skin.

Studies by Aggazzotti et al. (1990, 1993, 1995, 1998) showed that exposure to chlorinated swimming pool water and the air above swimming pools can lead to an increase in detectable THMs in both plasma and alveolar air, but the concentration in alveolar air rapidly falls after exiting the pool area (Tables 4.7 and 4.8).

2. Chloramines, chlorite and chlorate

Exposure to chloramines in the atmosphere of indoor pools was studied in France by Hery et al. (1995) in response to complaints of eye and respiratory tract irritation by pool attendants. They found concentrations of up to 0.84 mg/m^3 and that levels were generally higher in pools with recreational activities such as slides and fountains.

Erdinger et al. (1999) examined the concentrations of chlorite and chlorate in swimming pools and found that while chlorite was not detectable, chlorate concentrations varied from 1 mg/l to, in one extreme case, 40 mg/l. Strähle et al. (2000) found chlorate concentrations of up to 142 mg/l. The concentrations of chlorate in chlorine-disinfected pools were close to the limit of detection of 1 mg/l, but the mean concentration of chlorate in sodium hypochlorite-disinfected pools was about 17 mg/l. Chlorate concentrations were much lower in pools disinfected with hypochlorite and ozone, and the chlorate levels were related to the levels in hypochlorite stock solutions.

3. Other disinfection by-products

A number of other disinfection by-products have been examined in swimming pool water; these are summarized in Tables 4.9–4.11. Dichloroacetic acid has also been detected in swimming pool water. In a German study of 15 indoor and 3 outdoor swimming pools (Clemens & Scholer, 1992), dichloroacetic acid concentrations averaged 5.6 $\mu g/l$ and 119.9 $\mu g/l$ in indoor and outdoor pools, respectively. The mean concentration of dichloroacetic acid in three indoor pools in the USA was 419 $\mu g/l$ (Kim & Weisel, 1998). The difference between the results of these two studies may be due to differences in the amounts of chlorine used to disinfect swimming pools, sample collection time relative to chlorination of the water, or addition or exchanges of water in the pools.

Table 4.4. Concentrations of trihalomethanes measured in swimming pool water

Country	Chloroform Mean	Chloroform Range	BDCM Mean	BDCM Range	DBCM Mean	DBCM Range	Bromoform Mean	Bromoform Range	Pool type	Reference
				Disinfection by-product concentration (µg/l)						
Poland		35.9-99.7		2.3-14.7		0.2-0.8		0.2-203.2	indoor	Biziuk et al., 1993
Italy	93.7	19-94							indoor	Aggazzotti et al., 1993
	33.7	9-179							indoor	Aggazzotti et al., 1995
		25-43	2.3	1.8-2.8	0.8	0.5-10	0.1	0.1	indoor	Aggazzotti et al., 1998
USA	37.9								indoor	Copaken, 1990
		4-402		1-72		<0.1-8		<0.1-1	outdoor	Armstrong & Golden, 1986
		3-580		1-90		0.3-30		<0.1-60	indoor	
		<0.1-530		<0.1-105		<0.1-48		<0.1-183	hot tub	
Germany	14.6	2.4-29.8							indoor	Eichelsdörfer et al., 1981
	43	14.6-111							outdoor	
	198	43-980	22.6	0.1-150	10.9	0.1-140	1.8	<0.1-88	indoor	Lahl et al., 1981
		0.5-23.6		1.9-16.5		<0.1-3.4		<0.1-3.3	indoor	Ewers et al., 1987
		<0.1-32.9		<0.1-54.5		<0.1-1.0		<0.1-0.5	hydrotherapy	
		<0.1-0.9		<0.1-1.4		<0.1-16.4		2.4-132	hydrotherapy	
		3.6-82.1		1.6-17.3		<0.1-15.1		<0.1-4.0	outdoor	
	94.9	40.6-117.5	4.8	4.2-5.4	1.8	0.78-2.6			indoor	Puchert et al., 1989
	80.7		8.9		1.5		<0.1		indoor	Puchert, 1994
	74.9		11.0		3.0		0.23		outdoor	
		3-27.8		0.69-5.64		0.03-6.51		0.02-0.83	indoor	Cammann & Hübner, 1995
		1.8-28		1.3-3.4		<0.1-1	<0.1		indoor	Jovanovic et al., 1995
		8-11							indoor	Schössner & Koch, 1995
	14	0.51-69	2.5	0.12-15	0.59	0.03-4.9	0.16	<0.03-8.1	indoor	Stottmeister, 1998, 1999
	30	0.69-114	4.5	0.27-25	1.1	0.04-8.8	0.28	<0.03-3.4	outdoor	
	4.3	0.82-12	1.3	0.19-4.1	0.4	0.03-0.91	0.08	<0.03-0.22	hydrotherapy	
	3.8	6.4 (max.)							spa	Erdinger et al., 1997b
		7.1-24.8							indoor pool	Erdinger et al., 2004
Denmark		145-151							indoor	Kaas & Rudiengaard, 1987
Hungary	11.4	<2-62.3	2.9	<1.0-11.4					indoor	Borsányi, 1998
UK	121.1	45-212	8.3	2.5-23	2.7	0.67-7	0.9	0.67-2	indoor pools	Chu & Nieuwenhuijsen, 2002

BDCM = bromodichloromethane; DBCM = dibromochloromethane

4.5.2 Risks associated with disinfection by-products

The guideline values in the WHO *Guidelines for Drinking-water Quality* can be used to screen for potential risks arising from disinfection by-products from swimming pools and similar environments, while making appropriate allowance for the much lower quantities of water ingested, shorter exposure periods and non-ingestion exposure. Although there are data to indicate that the concentrations of chlorination by-products in swimming pools and similar environments may exceed the WHO guideline values for drinking-water (WHO, 2004), available evidence indicates that for reasonably well managed pools, concentrations less than the drinking-water guideline values can be consistently achieved. Since the drinking-water guidelines are intended to reflect tolerable risks over a lifetime, this provides an additional level of reassurance. Drinking-water guidelines assume an intake of 2 litres per day, but as considered above, ingestion of swimming pool water is considerably less than this; recent measured data (Section 4.1.1) indicate an extreme of about 100 ml (Evans et al., 2001). Uptake via skin absorption and inhalation (in the case of THMs) is proportionally greater than from drinking-water and is significant, but the low oral intake allows a margin that can, to an extent, account for this. Under such circumstances, the risks from exposure to chlorination by-products in reasonably well managed swimming pools would be considered to be small and must be set against the benefits of aerobic exercise and the risks of infectious disease in the absence of disinfection.

Levels of chlorate and chlorite in swimming pool water have not been extensively studied; however, in some cases, high chlorate concentrations have been reported, which greatly exceeded the WHO provisional drinking-water guideline (0.7 mg/l) and which would, for a child ingesting 100 ml of water, result in possible toxic effects. Exposure, therefore, needs to be minimized, with frequent dilution of pool water with fresh water, and care taken to ensure that chlorate levels do not build up in stored hypochlorite disinfectants.

The chloramines and bromamines, particularly nitrogen trichloride and nitrogen tribromide, which are both volatile (Holzwarth et al., 1984), can give rise to significant eye and respiratory irritation in swimmers and pool attendants (Massin et al., 1998). In addition, nitrogen trichloride has an intense and unpleasant odour at concentrations in water as low as 0.02 mg/l (Kirk & Othmer, 1993). Studies of subjects using swimming pools and non-swimming attendants have shown a number of changes and symptoms that appear to be associated with exposure to the atmosphere in swimming pools. Various authors have suggested that these were associated with nitrogen trichloride exposure in particular (Carbonnelle et al., 2002; Thickett et al., 2002; Bernard et al., 2003), although the studies were unable to confirm the specific chemicals that were the cause of the symptoms experienced. Symptoms are likely to be particularly pronounced in those suffering from asthma. Yoder et al. (2004) reported two incidents, between 2001 and 2002, where a total of 52 people were adversely affected by a build-up of chloramines in indoor pool water. One of the incidents related to a hotel pool, and 32 guests reported coughs, eye and throat irritation and difficulty in breathing. Both incidents were attributed to chloramines on the basis of the clinical syndrome and setting. Hery et al. (1995) found that complaints from non-swimmers were initiated at a concentration of 0.5 mg/m^3 chlorine species (expressed in units of nitrogen trichloride) in the atmosphere of indoor pools and hot tubs. It is recommended that 0.5 mg/m^3 would be suitable as a provisional value for chlorine species,

Table 4.5. Concentrations of trihalomethanes measured in the air above the pool water surface

Country	Chloroform		BDCM			DBCM			Bromoform		Pool type	Reference
	Mean	Range	Mean	Range		Mean	Range		Mean	Range		
Italy	214	66–650	19.5	5–100		6.6	0.1–14		0.2		indoor[1]	Aggazzotti et al., 1995
	140	49–280	17.4	2–58		13.3	4–30		0.2		indoor[1]	Aggazzotti et al., 1993
	169	35–195	20	16–24		11.4	9–14		0.2		indoor[1]	Aggazzotti et al., 1998
Canada		597–1630									indoor	Lévesque et al., 1994
Germany	65		9.2			3.8					indoor[1]	Jovanovic et al., 1995
	36		5.6			1.2					indoor[2]	
	5.6		0.21								outdoor[1]	
	2.3										outdoor[1]	
	3.3	0.33–9.7	0.4	0.08–2.0		0.1	0.02–0.5		<0.03		outdoor[1]	Stottmeister, 1998, 1999
	1.2	0.36–2.2	0.1	0.03–0.16		0.05	0.03–0.08		<0.03		outdoor[2]	
	39	5.6–206	4.9	0.85–16		0.9	0.05–3.2		0.1	<0.03–3.0	indoor[1]	
	30	1.7–136	4.1	0.23–13		0.8	0.05–2.9		0.08	<0.03–0.7	indoor[2]	
USA		<0.1–1		<0.1			<0.1			<0.1	outdoor[3]	Armstrong & Golden, 1986
		<0.1–260		<0.1–10			<0.1–5			<0.1–14	indoor[3]	
		<0.1–47		<0.1–10			<0.1–5			<0.1–14	hot tub[3]	

BDCM = bromodichloromethane; DBCM = dibromochloromethane
[a] Measured 20 cm above the water surface
[b] Measured 150 cm above the water surface
[c] Measured 200 cm above the water surface

Table 4.6. Comparison of trihalomethane concentrations in blood of swimmers after a 1-h swim, in pool water and in ambient air of indoor and outdoor pools[a]

	THM concentration (mean, range)	
	Indoor pool	Outdoor pool
Blood of swimmers (µg/l)	0.48 (0.23–0.88)	0.11 (<0.06–0.21)
Pool water (µg/l)	19.6 (4.5–45.8)	73.1 (3.2–146)
Air 20 cm above the water surface (µg/m³)	93.6 (23.9–179.9)	8.2 (2.1–13.9)
Air 150 cm above the water surface (µg/m³)	61.6 (13.4–147.1)	2.5 (<0.7–4.7)

[a] Adapted from Strähle et al., 2000

Table 4.7. Concentrations of trihalomethanes in plasma of 127 swimmers[a]

THM	No. positive/no. samples	Mean THM concentration (µg/l)	Range of THM concentrations (µg/l)
Chloroform	127/127	1.06	0.1–3.0
BDCM	25/127	0.14	<0.1–0.3
DBCM	17/127	0.1	<0.1–0.1

[a] Adapted from Aggazzotti et al., 1990

Table 4.8. Comparison of trihalomethane levels in ambient air and alveolar air in swimmers prior to arrival at the swimming pool, during swimming and after swimming[a]

	THM levels (µg/m³) at various monitoring times[b]				
	A	B	C	D	E
Chloroform					
Ambient air	20.7 ± 5.3	91.7 ± 15.4	169.7 ± 26.8	20.0 ± 8.4	19.2 ± 8.8
Alveolar air	9.3 ± 3.1	29.4 ± 13.3	76.5 ± 18.6	26.4 ± 4.9	19.1 ± 2.5
BDCM					
Ambient air	n.q.	10.5 ± 3.1	20.0 ± 4.1	n.q.	n.q.
Alveolar air	n.q.	2.7 ± 1.2	6.5 ± 1.3	2.7 ± 1.1	1.9 ± 1.1
DBCM					
Ambient air	n.q.	5.2 ± 1.5	11.4 ± 2.1	n.q.	n.q.
Alveolar air	n.q.	0.8 ± 0.8	1.4 ± 0.9	0.3 ± 0.2	0.20 ± 0.1
Bromoform					
Ambient air	n.q.	0.2	0.2	0.2	n.q.
Alveolar air	n.q.	n.q.	n.q.	n.q.	n.q.

[a] Adapted from Aggazzotti et al., 1998

[b] Five competitive swimmers (three males and two females) were monitored A: Prior to arrival at the pool; B: After 1 h resting at poolside before swimming; C: After a 1-h swim; D: 1 h after swimming had stopped; and E: 1.5 h after swimming had stopped. D and E occurred after departing the pool area. n.q. = not quantified

Table 4.9. Concentrations of haloacetic acids measured in swimming pool water

Country	MCAA		MBAA		DCAA		DBAA		TCAA		Pool type	Reference
	Mean	Range	Mean	Range	Mean	Range	Mean	Range	Mean	Range		
Germany	26	2.6–81	0.32	<0.5–3.3	23	1.5–192	0.57	<0.2–7.7	42	3.5–199	indoor	Stottmeister & Naglitsch, 1996
	32	2.5–174	0.15	<0.5–1.9	8.8	1.8–27	0.64	<0.2–4.8	15	1.1–45	hydrotherapy	
	26	2.5–112	0.06	<0.5–1.7	132	6.2–562	0.08	<0.2–1.3	249	8.2–887	outdoor	
									30		hot tub	Lahl et al., 1984
										25–136	indoor	
										2.3–100	indoor	Mannschott et al., 1995

MCAA = monochloroacetic acid; MBAA = monobromoacetic acid; DCAA = dichloroacetic acid; DBAA = dibromoacetic acid; TCAA = trichloroacetic acid

Table 4.10. Concentrations of haloacetonitriles measured in swimming pool water

Country	DCAN		DBAN		TCAN		Pool type	Reference
	Mean	Range	Mean	Range	Mean	Range		
Germany		6.7–18.2					indoor	Puchert, 1994
		<0.5–2.5					outdoor	
	13	0.13–148	2.3	<0.01–24	1.7	<0.01–11	indoor	Stottmeister, 1998, 1999
	9.9	0.22–57	0.62	<0.01–2.8	1.5	<0.01–7.8	hydrotherapy	
	45	<0.01–0.02	2.5	<0.01–16	1.3	<0.01–10	outdoor	
	24		49				indoor	Baudisch et al., 1997
							seawater	

DCAN = dichloroacetonitrile; DBAN = dibromoacetonitrile; TCAN = trichloroacetonitrile

Table 4.11. Concentrations of chloropicrin, chloral hydrate and bromal hydrate measured in swimming pool water

Country	Chloropicrin		Chloral hydrate		Bromal hydrate		Pool type	Reference
	Mean	Range	Mean	Range	Mean	Range		
Germany		0.1–2.6					indoor	Schöler & Schopp, 1984
		0.32–0.8					indoor	Puchert, 1994
		<0.01–0.75					outdoor	Stottmeister, 1998, 1999
	0.32	0.03–1.6					indoor	
	0.20	0.04–0.78					hydrotherapy	
	1.3	0.01–10					outdoor	
			265				indoor	Baudisch et al., 1997
					230		seawater	Baudisch et al., 1997
				0.5–104			indoor	Mannschott et al., 1995

expressed as nitrogen trichloride, in the atmosphere of indoor swimming pools and similar environments. However, more specific data are needed on the potential for exacerbation of asthma in affected individuals, since this is a significant proportion of the population in some countries. There is also a potential issue regarding those that are very frequent pool users and who may be exposed for longer periods per session, such as competitive swimmers. It is particularly important that the management of pools used for such purposes is optimized in order to reduce the potential for exposure (Section 5.9).

4.6 Risks associated with plant and equipment malfunction

Chemical hazards can arise from malfunction of plant and associated equipment. This hazard can be reduced, if not eliminated, through proper installation and effective routine maintenance programmes. The use of gas detection systems and automatic shutdown can also be an effective advance warning of plant malfunction. The use of remote monitoring is becoming more commonplace in after-hours response to plant and equipment malfunction or shutdown.

4.7 References

Aggazzotti G, Fantuzzi G, Tartoni PL, Predieri G (1990) Plasma chloroform concentration in swimmers using indoor swimming pools. *Archives of Environmental Health,* 45A(3): 175–179.

Aggazzotti G, Fantuzzi G, Righi E, Tartoni PL, Cassinadri T, Predieri G (1993) Chloroform in alveolar air of individuals attending indoor swimming pools. *Archives of Environmental Health*, 48: 250–254.

Aggazzotti G, Fantuzzi G, Righi E, Predieri G (1995) Environmental and biological monitoring of chloroform in indoor swimming pools. *Journal of Chromatography*, A710: 181–190.

Aggazzotti G, Fantuzzi G, Righi E, Predieri G (1998) Blood and breath analyses as biological indicators of exposure to trihalomethanes in indoor swimming pools. *Science of the Total Environment*, 217: 155–163.

Armstrong DW, Golden T (1986) Determination of distribution and concentration of trihalomethanes in aquatic recreational and therapeutic facilities by electron-capture GC. *LC-GC*, 4: 652–655.

Baudisch C, Pansch G, Prösch J, Puchert W (1997) [*Determination of volatile halogenated hydrocarbons in chlorinated swimming pool water. Research report.*] Außenstelle Schwerin, Landeshygieneinstitut Mecklenburg-Vorpommern (in German).

Bernard A, Carbonnelle S, Michel O, Higuet S, de Burbure C, Buchet J-P, Hermans C, Dumont X, Doyle I (2003) Lung hyperpermeability and asthma prevalence in schoolchildren: unexpected associations with the attendance in indoor chlorinated swimming pools. *Occupational and Environmental Medicine*, 60: 385–394.

Biziuk M, Czerwinski J, Kozlowski E (1993) Identification and determination of organohalogen compounds in swimming pool water. *International Journal of Environmental Analytical Chemistry*, 46: 109–115.

Borsányi M (1998) *THMs in Hungarian swimming pool waters.* Budapest, National Institute of Environmental Health, Department of Water Hygiene (unpublished).

Cammann K, Hübner K (1995) Trihalomethane concentrations in swimmers' and bath attendants' blood and urine after swimming or working in indoor swimming pools. *Archives of Environmental Health*, 50: 61–65.

Carbonnelle S, Francaux M, Doyle I, Dumont X, de Burbure C, Morel G, Michel O, Bernard A (2002) Changes in serum pneumoproteins caused by short-term exposures to nitrogen trichloride in indoor chlorinated swimming pools. *Biomarkers*, 7(6): 464–478.

Chu H, Nieuwenhuijsen MJ (2002) Distribution and determinants of trihalomethane concentrations in indoor swimming pools. *Occupational and Environmental Medicine*, 59: 243–247.

Clemens M, Scholer HF (1992) Halogenated organic compounds in swimming pool waters. *Zentralblatt für Hygiene und Umweltmedizin*, 193(1): 91–98.

Copaken J (1990) Trihalomethanes: Is swimming pool water hazardous? In: Jolley RL, Condie LW, Johnson JD, Katz S, Minear RA, Mattice JS, Jacobs VA, eds. *Water chlorination. Vol. 6*. Chelsea, MI, Lewis Publishers, pp. 101–106.

Eichelsdörfer D, Jandik J, Weil L (1981) [Formation and occurrence of organic halogenated compounds in swimming pool water.] *A.B. Archiv des Badewesens*, 34: 167–172 (in German).

Erdinger L, Kirsch F, Sonntag H-G (1997a) [Potassium as an indicator of anthropogenic contamination of swimming pool water.] *Zentralblatt für Hygiene und Umweltmedizin*, 200(4): 297–308 (in German).

Erdinger L, Kirsch F, Hoppner A, Sonntag H-G (1997b) Haloforms in hot spring pools. *Zentralblatt für Hygiene und Umweltmedizin*. 200: 309–317 (in German).

Erdinger L, Kirsch F, Sonntag H-G (1999) Chlorate as an inorganic disinfection by-product in swimming pools. *Zentralblatt für Hygiene und Umweltmedizin*, 202: 61–75.

Erdinger L, Kuhn KP, Kirsch F, Feldhues R, Frobel T, Nohynek B, Gabrio T (2004) Pathways of trihalomethane uptake in swimming pools. *International Journal of Hygiene and Environmental Health*, 207: 1–5.

Evans O, Cantú R, Bahymer TD, Kryak DD, Dufour AP (2001) *A pilot study to determine the water volume ingested by recreational swimmers*. Paper presented to 2001 Annual Meeting of the Society for Risk Analysis, Seattle, Washington, 2–5 December 2001.

Ewers H, Hajimiragha H, Fischer U, Böttger A, Ante R (1987) [Organic halogenated compounds in swimming pool waters.] *Forum Städte-Hygiene*, 38: 77–79 (in German).

Fantuzzi G, Righi E, Predieri G, Ceppelli G, Gobba F, Aggazzotti G (2001) Occupational exposure to trihalomethanes in indoor swimming pools. *Science of the Total Environment*, 17: 257–265.

Grguric G, Trefry JH, Keaffaber JJ (1994) Ozonation products of bromine and chlorine in seawater aquaria. *Water Research*, 28: 1087–1094.

Gundermann KO, Jentsch F, Matthiessen A (1997) [*Final report on the research project "Trihalogenmethanes in indoor seawater and saline pools"*.] Kiel, Institut für Hygiene und Umweltmedizin der Universität Kiel (in German).

Gunkel K, Jessen H-J (1988) [The problem of urea in bathing water.] *Zeitschrift für die Gesamte Hygiene*, 34: 248–250 (in German).

Hery M, Hecht G, Gerber JM, Gendree JC, Hubert G, Rebuffaud J (1995) Exposure to chloramines in the atmosphere of indoor swimming pools. *Annals of Occupational Hygiene*, 39: 427–439.

Holzwarth G, Balmer RG, Soni L (1984) The fate of chlorine and chloramines in cooling towers. *Water Research*, 18: 1421–1427.

Isaak RA, Morris JC (1980) Rates of transfer of active chlorine between nitrogenous substrates. In: Jolley RL, ed. *Water chlorination. Vol. 3*. Ann Arbor, MI, Ann Arbor Science Publishers.

Jandik J (1977) [*Studies on decontamination of swimming pool water with consideration of ozonation of nitrogen containing pollutants*.] Dissertation. Munich, Technical University Munich (in German).

JECFA (2004) *Evaluation of certain food additives and contaminants*. Sixty-first report of the Joint FAO/WHO Expert Committee on Food Additives (WHO Technical Report Series No. 922).

Jovanovic S, Wallner T, Gabrio T (1995) [*Final report on the research project "Presence of haloforms in pool water, air and in swimmers and lifeguards in outdoor and indoor pools"*.] Stuttgart, Landesgesundheitsamt Baden-Württemberg (in German).

Judd SJ, Bullock G (2003) The fate of chlorine and organic materials in swimming pools. *Chemosphere*, 51(9): 869–879.

Kaas P, Rudiengaard P (1987) [*Toxicologic and epidemiologic aspects of organochlorine compounds in bathing water*.] Paper presented to the 3rd Symposium on "Problems of swimming pool water hygiene", Reinhardsbrunn (in German).

Kelsall HL, Sim MR (2001) Skin irritation in users of brominated pools. *International Journal of Environmental Health Research,* 11: 29–40.

Kim H, Weisel CP (1998) Dermal absorption of dichloro- and trichloroacetic acids from chlorinated water. *Journal of Exposure Analysis and Environmental Epidemiology,* 8(4): 555–575.

Kirk RE, Othmer DF (1993) *Encyclopedia of chemical technology,* 4th ed. *Vol. 5.* New York, NY, John Wiley & Sons, p. 916.

Lahl U, Bätjer K, Duszeln JV, Gabel B, Stachel B, Thiemann W (1981) Distribution and balance of volatile halogenated hydrocarbons in the water and air of covered swimming pools using chlorine for water disinfection. *Water Research,* 15: 803–814.

Lahl U, Stachel B, Schröer W, Zeschmar B (1984) [Determination of organohalogenic acids in water samples.] *Zeitschrift für Wasser- und Abwasser-Forschung,* 17: 45–49 (in German).

Latta D (1995) Interference in a melamine-based determination of cyanuric acid concentration. *Journal of the Swimming Pool and Spa Industry,* 1(2): 37–39.

Lévesque B, Ayotte P, LeBlanc A, Dewailly E, Prud'Homme D, Lavoie R, Allaire S, Levallois P (1994) Evaluation of dermal and respiratory chloroform exposure in humans. *Environmental Health Perspectives,* 102: 1082–1087.

Mannschott P, Erdinger L, Sonntag H-P (1995) [Determination of halogenated organic compounds in swimming pool water.] *Zentralblatt für Hygiene und Umweltmedizin,* 197: 516–533 (in German).

Massin N, Bohadana AB, Wild P, Héry M, Toamain JP, Hubert G (1998) Respiratory symptoms and bronchial responsiveness in lifeguards exposed to nitrogen trichloride in indoor swimming pools. *Occupational and Environmental Medicine,* 55: 258–263.

MDHSS (undated) *Swimming pool and spa water chemistry.* Missouri Department of Health and Senior Services, Section for Environmental Health (http://www.health.state.mo.us/RecreationalWater/PoolSpaChem.pdf).

Puchert W (1994) [*Determination of volatile halogenated hydrocarbons in different environmental compartments as basis for the estimation of a possible pollution in West Pommerania.*] Dissertation. Bremen, University of Bremen (in German).

Puchert W, Prösch J, Köppe F-G, Wagner H (1989) [Occurrence of volatile halogenated hydrocarbons in bathing water.] *Acta Hydrochimica et Hydrobiologica,* 17: 201–205 (in German).

Rakestraw LF (1994) *A comprehensive study on disinfection conditions in public swimming pools in Pinellas County, Florida.* Study conducted by Pinellas County Public Health Unit and The Occidental Chemical Corporation. Presented on behalf of the Pool Study Team at the NSPI International Expo, New Orleans.

Raykar PV, Fung MC, Anderson BD (1988) The role of protein and lipid domains in the uptake of solutes by human stratum corneum. *Pharmacological Research,* 5(3): 140–150.

Rycroft RJ, Penny PT (1983) Dermatoses associated with brominated swimming pools. *British Medical Journal,* 287(6390): 462.

Sandel BB (1990) *Disinfection by-products in swimming pools and spas.* Olin Corporation Research Center (Report CNHC-RR-90-154) (available from Arch Chemical, Charleston).

Schöler HF, Schopp D (1984) [Volatile halogenated hydrocarbons in swimming pool waters.] *Forum Städte-Hygiene,* 35: 109–112 (in German).

Schössner H, Koch A (1995) [Investigations of trihalogenmethane-concentrations in swimming pool water.] *Forum Städte-Hygiene,* 46: 354–357 (in German).

Stottmeister E (1998) *Disinfection by-products in German swimming pool waters.* Paper presented to 2nd International Conference on Pool Water Quality and Treatment, 4 March 1998, School of Water Sciences, Cranfield University, Cranfield, UK.

Stottmeister E (1999) [Occurrence of disinfection by-products in swimming pool waters.] *Umweltmedizinischer Informationsdienst,* 2: 21–29 (in German).

Stottmeister E, Naglitsch F (1996) [*Human exposure to other disinfection by-products than trihalomethanes in swimming pools.*] Annual report of the Federal Environmental Agency, Berlin, Germany (in German).

Strähle J, Sacre C, Schwenk M, Jovanovic S, Gabrio T, Lustig B (2000) [*Risk assessment of exposure of swimmers to disinfection by-products formed in swimming pool water treatment.*] Final report on the research project of DVGW 10/95, Landesgesundheitsamt Baden-Württemberg, Stuttgart (in German).

Taras MJ (1953) Effect of free residual chlorination on nitrogen compounds in water. *Journal of the American Water Works Association*, 45: 4761.

Thickett KM, McCoach JS, Gerber JM, Sadhra S, Burge PS (2002) Occupational asthma caused by chloramines in indoor swimming-pool air. *European Respiratory Journal,* 19(5): 827–832.

WHO (1999) *Principles for the assessment of risks to human health from exposure to chemicals.* Geneva, World Health Organization (Environmental Health Criteria 210).

WHO (2000) *Disinfectants and disinfectant by-products.* Geneva, World Health Organization (Environmental Health Criteria 216).

WHO (2004) *Guidelines for drinking-water quality*, 3rd ed. *Vol. 1. Recommendations.* Geneva, World Health Organization.

Yoder JS, Blackburn BG, Craun GF, Hill V, Levy DA, Chen N, Lee SH, Calderon RL, Beach MJ (2004) Surveillance of waterborne-disease outbreaks associated with recreational water – United States, 2001–2002. *Morbidity and Mortality Weekly Report*, 53(SS08): 1–22.

CHAPTER 5
Managing water and air quality

This chapter builds upon the background provided in Chapters 2, 3 and 4 and provides guidance relating to water and air quality management (risk management specific to certain microbial hazards is covered in greater detail in Chapter 3). The primary water and air quality health challenges to be dealt with are, in typical order of public health priority:

- controlling clarity to minimize injury hazard;
- controlling water quality to prevent the transmission of infectious disease; and
- controlling potential hazards from disinfection by-products.

All of these challenges can be met through a combination of the following factors:

- treatment (to remove particulates, pollutants and microorganisms), including filtration and disinfection (to remove/inactivate infectious microorganisms);
- pool hydraulics (to ensure effective distribution of disinfectant throughout the pool, good mixing and removal of contaminated water);
- addition of fresh water at frequent intervals (to dilute substances that cannot be removed from the water by treatment);
- cleaning (to remove biofilms from surfaces, sediments from the pool floor and particulates adsorbed to filter materials); and
- ventilation of indoor pools (to remove volatile disinfection by-products and radon).

Controlling clarity, the most important water quality criterion, involves adequate water treatment, including filtration. The control of pathogens is typically achieved by a combination of circulation of pool water through treatment (normally requiring some form of filtration plus disinfection) and the application of a chemical residual disinfectant to inactivate microorganisms introduced to the pool itself by, for instance, bathers. As not all infectious agents are killed by the most frequently used residual disinfectants, and as circulation through the physical treatment processes is slow, it is necessary to minimize accidental faecal releases and vomit (and to respond effectively to them when they occur) and to minimize the introduction of bather-shed organisms by pre-swim hygiene. Microbial colonization of surfaces can be a problem and is generally controlled through adequate levels of cleaning and disinfection. The control of disinfection by-products requires dilution, selection of source waters without DBP precursors (may include water pretreatment if necessary), pre-swim showering, treatment, disinfection modification or optimization and bather education.

Figure 5.1 outlines the components and shows a general layout of a 'typical' pool treatment system. Most pools have a pumped system and water is kept in continuous

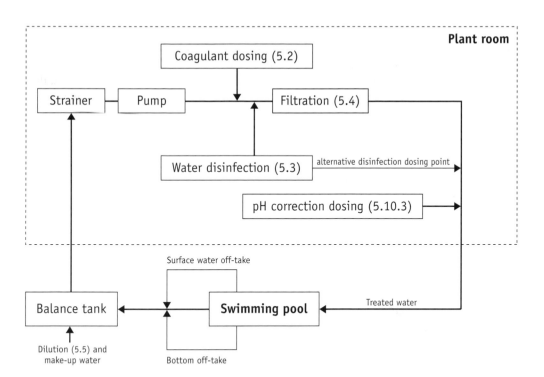

Figure 5.1. Water treatment processes in a 'typical pool' (relevant section numbers are identified in parentheses)

circulation (see Section 5.6), with fresh water being added for dilution of materials that are not effectively removed by treatment and to account for losses (often referred to as make-up water).

5.1 Pre-swim hygiene

In some countries, it is common to shower before a swim. Showering will help to remove traces of sweat, urine, faecal matter, cosmetics, suntan oil and other potential water contaminants. Where pool users normally shower before swimming, pool water is cleaner, easier to disinfect with smaller amounts of chemicals and thus more pleasant to swim in. Money is saved on chemicals (offset to some extent by the extra cost of heating shower water, where necessary). The most appropriate setup for showers (e.g. private to encourage nude showering, a continuously run or automatic 'tunnel' arrangement) will vary according to country, but pool owners and managers should actively encourage showering. Showers must run to waste and should be managed to control *Legionella* growth (see Chapter 3).

The role of footbaths and showers in dealing with papillomavirus and foot infections is under question. However, it is generally accepted that there must be some barrier between outdoor dirt and the pool in order to minimize the transfer of dirt into the pool. A foot spray is probably the best of the alternatives to footbaths. Where outdoor footwear is allowed poolside (e.g. some outdoor pools), separate poolside drainage systems can minimize the transfer of pollutants to the pool water.

Toilets should be provided and located where they can be conveniently used before entering and after leaving the pool. All users should be encouraged to use the toilets before bathing to minimize urination in the pool and accidental faecal releases. If babies and toddlers (that are not toilet trained) are allowed in the pool facilities, they should, wherever possible, wear leak-proof swimwear (that will contain any urine or faecal release) and, ideally, they should have access only to small pools that can be completely drained if an accidental faecal release occurs.

5.2 Coagulation

Coagulants (or flocculants) enhance the removal of dissolved, colloidal or suspended material by bringing it out of solution or suspension as solids (coagulation), then clumping the solids together (flocculation), producing a floc, which is more easily trapped during filtration. Coagulants are particularly important in helping to remove the oocysts and cysts of *Cryptosporidium* and *Giardia* (Pool Water Treatment Advisorz Group, pers. comm.; Gregory, 2002), which otherwise may pass through the filter. Coagulant efficiency is dependent upon pH, which, therefore, needs to be controlled.

5.3 Disinfection

Disinfection is part of the treatment process whereby pathogenic microorganisms are inactivated by chemical (e.g. chlorination) or physical (e.g. UV radiation) means such that they represent no significant risk of infection. Circulating pool water is disinfected during the treatment process, and the entire water body is disinfected by the application of a residual disinfectant (chlorine- or bromine-based), which partially inactivates agents added to the pool by bathers. Facilities that are difficult or impossible to disinfect pose a special set of problems and generally require very high rates of dilution to maintain water quality. For disinfection to occur with any biocidal chemical, the oxidant demand of the water being treated must be satisfied and sufficient chemical must remain to effect disinfection.

5.3.1 Choosing a disinfectant

Issues to be considered in the choice of a disinfectant and application system include:

- safety (while occupational health and safety are not specifically covered in this volume, operator safety is an important factor to consider);
- compatibility with the source water (it is necessary to either match the disinfectant to the pH of the source water or adjust the source water pH);
- type and size of pool (e.g. disinfectant may be more readily degraded or lost through evaporation in outdoor pools);
- ability to remain in water as residual after application;
- bathing load; and
- operation of the pool (i.e. capacity and skills for supervision and management).

The disinfectant used as part of swimming pool water treatment should ideally meet the following criteria:

- effective and rapid inactivation of pathogenic microorganisms;
- capacity for ongoing oxidation to assist in the control of all contaminants during pool use;

- a wide margin between effective biocidal concentration and concentrations resulting in adverse effects on human health (adverse health effects of disinfectants and disinfection by-products are reviewed in Chapter 4);
- availability of a quick and easy measurement of the disinfectant concentration in pool water (simple analytical test methods and equipment); and
- potential to measure the disinfectant concentration online to permit automatic control of disinfectant dosing and continuous recording of the values measured.

5.3.2 Characteristics of various disinfectants

1. Chlorine-based disinfectants

Chlorination is the most widely used pool water disinfection method, usually in the form of chlorine gas, a hypochlorite salt (sodium, calcium, lithium) or chlorinated isocyanurates. While chlorine gas can be safely and effectively used, it does have the potential to cause serious health impacts, and care must be taken to ensure that health concerns do not arise.

When chlorine gas or hypochlorite is added to water, hypochlorous acid (HOCl) is formed. Hypochlorous acid dissociates in water into its constituents H^+ and OCl^- (hypochlorite ion), as follows:

$$HOCl \quad \leftrightarrow \quad H^+ \quad + \quad OCl^-$$

$$\text{hypochlorous} \qquad \text{hydrogen} \qquad \text{hypochlorite}$$
$$\text{acid} \qquad\qquad \text{ion} \qquad\qquad \text{ion}$$

The degree of dissociation depends on pH and (much less) on temperature. Dissociation is minimal at pH levels below 6. At pH levels of 6.5–8.5, a change occurs from undissociated hypochlorous acid to nearly complete dissociation. Hypochlorous acid is a much stronger disinfectant than hypochlorite ion. At a pH of 8.0, 21% of the free chlorine exists in the hypochlorous acid form (acting as a strong, fast, oxidizing disinfectant), while at a pH of 8.5, only 12% of that chlorine exists as hypochlorous acid. For this reason, the pH value should be kept relatively low and within defined limits (7.2–7.8 – see Section 5.10.3). Together, hypochlorous acid and OCl^- are referred to as free chlorine. The usual test for chlorine detects both free and total chlorine; to determine the effectiveness of disinfection, the pH value must also be known.

The chlorinated isocyanurate compounds are white crystalline compounds with a slight chlorine-type odour that provide free chlorine (as hypochlorous acid) when dissolved in water but which serve to provide a source of chlorine that is more resistant to the effects of UV light. They are widely used in outdoor or lightly loaded pools. They are an indirect source of chlorine, and the reaction is represented by the equation:

$$Cl_xH_{3-x}Cy \quad + \quad H_2O \quad \leftrightarrow \quad C_3H_3N_3O \quad + \quad HOCl$$

$$\text{chloroiso-} \qquad\quad \text{water} \qquad\qquad \text{cyanuric} \qquad \text{hypochlorous}$$
$$\text{cyanurates} \qquad\qquad\qquad\qquad\quad \text{acid} \qquad\qquad \text{acid}$$

$$x = 1 \text{ (mono-)}; 2 \text{ (di-)}; 3 \text{ (tri-)}$$

Free chlorine, cyanuric acid and chlorinated isocyanurate exist in equilibrium. The relative amounts of each compound are determined by the pH and free chlorine

---

concentration. As the disinfectant (HOCl) is used up, more chlorine atoms are released from the chloroisocyanurates to form hypochlorous acid. This results in an enrichment of cyanuric acid in the pool that cannot be removed by the water treatment process. Dilution with fresh water is necessary to keep the cyanuric acid concentration at a satisfactory level.

The balance between free chlorine and the level of cyanuric acid is critical and can be difficult to maintain. If the balance is lost because cyanuric acid levels become too high, unsatisfactory microbial conditions can result. Cyanuric acid in chlorinated water (whether introduced separately or present through the use of chlorinated isocyanurates) will reduce the amount of free chlorine. At low levels of cyanuric acid, there is very little effect; as the cyanuric acid level increases, however, the disinfecting and oxidizing properties of the free chlorine become progressively reduced. High levels of cyanuric acid cause a situation known as 'chlorine lock', when even very high levels of chlorine become totally locked with the cyanuric acid (stabilizer) and unavailable as disinfectant; however, this does not occur below cyanuric acid levels of 200 mg/l. It means, however, that the cyanuric acid level must be monitored and controlled relative to chlorine residual, and it is recommended that cyanurate levels should not exceed 100 mg/l. A simple turbidity test, where the degree of turbidity, following addition of the test chemical, is proportional to the cyanuric acid concentration, can be used to monitor levels. For effective disinfection, the pH value must also be monitored, because the influence of pH on disinfection efficiency is the same as described for chlorine as a disinfectant.

2. Bromine-based disinfectants

Elemental bromine is a heavy, dark red-brown, volatile liquid with fumes that are toxic and irritating to eyes and respiratory tract, and it is not considered suitable for swimming pool disinfection.

Bromine combines with some water impurities to form combined bromine, including bromamines. However, combined bromine acts as a disinfectant and produces less sharp and offensive odours than corresponding chloramines. Bromine does not oxidize ammonia and nitrogen compounds. Because of this, bromine cannot be used for shock dosing. When bromine disinfectants are used, shock dosing with chlorine is often necessary to oxidize ammonia and nitrogen compounds that eventually build up in the water (MDHSS, undated). Hypobromous acid reacts with sunlight and cannot be protected from the effects of UV light by cyanuric acid or other chemicals, and thus it is more practical to use bromine disinfectants for indoor pools.

For pool disinfection, bromine compounds are usually available in two forms, both of which are solids:

- a one-part system that is a compound (bromochlorodimethylhydantoin – BCDMH) of both bromine and chlorine, each attached to a nitrogen atom of dimethylhydantoin (DMH) as organic support for the halogens; and
- a two-part system that uses a bromide salt dissolved in water, activated by addition of a separate oxidizer.

BCDMH is an organic compound that dissolves in water to release hypobromous acid (HOBr) and hypochlorous acid. The latter reacts with bromide (Br⁻) (formed by a reduction of hypobromous acid) to form more hypobromous acid:

$$\text{Br-(DMH)-Cl} \quad + \quad 2\,H_2O \quad \leftrightarrow \quad HOBr \quad + \quad HOCl \quad + \quad \text{H-(DMH)-H}$$

bromochloro-	water	hypo-	hypochlorous	dimethyl-
dimethyl-		bromous	acid	hydantoin
hydantoin		acid		

disinfection
$$HOBr \quad \longrightarrow \quad Br^-$$
oxidation
$$HOCl + Br^- \quad \longrightarrow \quad HOBr + Cl^-$$

It can, therefore, be used both for treatment (oxidation) and to provide a residual disinfectant. Like the chlorinated isocyanurates, failure to maintain the correct relationship between the disinfectant residual and the organic component can result in unsatisfactory microbial conditions. The level of dimethylhydantoin in the water must be limited and should not exceed 200 mg/l. There is no poolside test kit available, and the need to regularly monitor dimethylhydantoin by a qualified laboratory is a disadvantage of the use of BCDMH. On the other hand, BCDMH is relatively innocuous in storage, is easy to dose and often does not need pH correction (as it is nearly neutral and has little effect on the pH values of most water). It is mostly available as tablets, cartridges or packets. BCDMH has a long shelf life and dissolves very slowly, so it may be used in floating and erosion-type feeders.

The two-part bromine system consists of a bromide salt (sodium bromide) and an oxidizer (hypochlorite, ozone). The sodium bromide is dosed to the water, passing through the treatment processes, upstream of the oxidizer, which is added to activate the bromide into hypobromous acid:

$$Br^- + \text{oxidizer} \quad \longrightarrow \quad HOBr$$

Disinfectant action returns hypobromous acid to bromide ions, which can again be reactivated. The pH value should be between 7.8 and 8.0 using this disinfection system (see also Section 5.10.3).

3. Ozone

Ozone can be viewed as the most powerful oxidizing and disinfecting agent that is available for pool water treatment (Rice, 1995; Saunus, 1998); it is generated on site and is potentially hazardous, particularly to the plant room operators. It is unsuitable for use as a residual disinfectant, as it readily vaporizes, is toxic and is heavier than air, leading to discomfort and adverse health effects (Locher, 1996). Ozonation is, therefore, followed by deozonation and addition of a residual disinfectant (i.e. chlorine- or bromine-based disinfectants).

All of the circulating water is treated with sufficient amounts of ozone (between 0.8 and 1.5 g/m^3, depending on the water temperature) to satisfy the oxidant demand of the water and attain a residual of dissolved ozone for several minutes. Under these conditions, ozone oxidizes many impurities (e.g. trihalomethane [THM] precursors) and microorganisms (disinfection), thereby reducing subsequent residual disinfectant requirements within the pool water. Lower disinfectant demand allows the pool operator to achieve the desired residual with a lower applied chlorine (or bromine) dose. As ozone can be inhaled by pool users and staff, excess ozone must be destroyed (forming oxygen and carbon dioxide) by deozonation (using granular activated carbon, activated heat-treated anthracite or thermal destruction), and an ozone leakage detector should be installed in the plant room. As residual disinfectants would also be removed by the deozonation process, they are, therefore, added after this. Microbial colonization of the deozonation media (especially granular activated carbon) can occur; this can be avoided by ensuring that there is residual disinfectant in the incoming water stream from the pool, maintaining the correct filter bed depth and an appropriate filter velocity.

Chloramines are oxidized by ozone into chloride and nitrate (Eichelsdörfer & Jandik, 1979, 1984), and precursors of disinfection by-products are also destroyed, resulting in very low levels of THMs (<0.02 mg/l) (Eichelsdörfer et al., 1981; Eichelsdörfer, 1987) and other chlorinated organics. The use of ozone in conjunction with chlorine (to ensure a residual disinfectant throughout the pool or similar environment) is, however, considerably more expensive than that of chlorine alone.

An ozone system in combination with BCDMH is also in use. However, the practice is to add only small amounts of ozone to this system to oxidize only the bromide (resulting from the spent hypobromous acid) back to hypobromous acid. Therefore, this BCDMH/ozone combination allows less BCDMH to be added. Ozone can also be used in combination with sodium bromide, as described above, as an oxidizer.

4. Ultraviolet (UV) radiation

Like ozone, the UV radiation process purifies the circulating water, without leaving a residual disinfectant. It inactivates microorganisms and breaks down some pollutants (e.g. chloramines) by photo-oxidation, decreasing the oxidant demand of the purified water.

UV disinfection can be achieved by UV irradiation at wavelengths between 200 and 300 nm. The following criteria are important in the selection of an appropriate UV system:

- type of microorganisms to be destroyed;
- water flow rate to be treated;
- type of lamps (low or medium pressure);
- UV dose;
- water temperature; and
- rate of disinfection.

For UV to be most effective, the water must be pretreated to remove turbidity-causing particulate matter that prevents the penetration of the UV radiation or absorbs the UV energy (Saunus, 1998). The UV lamps need to be cleaned periodically, as substances that build up on the lamps will reduce their pathogen inactivation efficiency over time. As with ozone, it is also necessary to use a chlorine- or bromine-based disinfectant to provide a residual disinfectant in the pool.

5. Algicides

Algicides are used to control algal growths, especially in outdoor pools. Algal growth is possible only if the nutrients phosphate, nitrogen and potassium are present in the pool water. Phosphate can be removed from the pool water by good coagulation and filtration during water treatment. Algal growth is best controlled by ensuring effective coagulation/filtration and good hydraulic design. In such properly managed swimming pools, the use of algicidal chemicals for the control of algae is not necessary (Gansloser et al., 1999). If problems persist, however, then proprietary algicides can be used. Quaternary ammonium and polyoximino compounds and copper salts can be used, but any based on mercury (a cumulative toxic heavy metal) should not be added to swimming pools. All should be used in strict accordance with the suppliers' instructions and should be intended for swimming pool use.

5.3.3 Disinfection by-products (DBP)

The production of disinfection by-products (see Chapter 4) can be controlled to a significant extent by minimizing the introduction of precursors though source water selection, good bather hygienic practices (e.g. pre-swim showering – see Section 5.1), maximizing their removal by well managed pool water treatment and replacement of water by the addition of fresh supplies (i.e. dilution of chemicals that cannot be removed). It is inevitable, however, that some volatile disinfection by-products, such as chloroform and nitrogen trichloride (a chloramine), may be produced in the pool water (depending upon the disinfection system used) and escape into the air. While levels of production should be minimized, this hazard can also be managed to some extent through good ventilation (see also Section 5.9).

5.3.4 Disinfectant dosing

The method of introducing disinfectants to the pool water influences their effectiveness, and, as illustrated in Figure 5.1, disinfectant dosing may occur pre- or post-filtration. Individual disinfectants have their own specific dosing requirements, but the following principles apply to all:

- Automatic dosing is preferable: electronic sensors monitor pH and residual disinfectant levels continuously and adjust the dosing correspondingly to maintain correct levels. Regular verification of the system (including manual tests on pool water samples) and good management are important. Section 5.10 describes the monitoring procedures.
- Hand-dosing (i.e. putting chemicals directly into the pool) is rarely justified. Manual systems of dosing must be backed up by good management of operation and monitoring. If manual dosing is employed, it is important that the pool is empty of bathers until the chemical has dispersed.
- Dosing pumps should be designed to shut themselves off if the circulation system fails (although automatic dosing monitors should remain in operation) to ensure that chemical dispersion is interrupted. If chemical dosing continues without water circulating, then high local concentrations of the dosed chemical will occur. On resumption of the circulation system, the high concentration will progress to the pool. If, for example, both hypochlorite and acid have been so dosed, the resultant mix containing chlorine gas may be dangerous to pool users.
- Residual disinfectants are generally dosed at the end of the treatment process. The treatment methods of coagulation, filtration and ozonation or ultraviolet serve to clarify the water, reduce the organic load (including precursors for the formation of disinfection by-products) and greatly reduce the microbial content, so that the post-treatment disinfection can be more effective and the amount of disinfectant required is minimized.

- It is important that disinfectants and pH-adjusting chemicals are well mixed with the water at the point of dosing.
- Dosing systems, like circulation, should operate 24 h a day.

Shock dosing

- Using a shock dose of chlorine as a preventive measure or to correct specific problems may be part of a strategy of proper pool management. Shock dosing is used to control a variety of pathogens and nuisance microorganisms and to destroy organic contaminants and chloramine compounds. Destroying chloramines requires free chlorine levels at least 10 times the level of combined chlorine. As a preventive measure, routine shock dosing (which is practised in some countries) typically involves raising free chlorine levels to at least 10 mg/l for between 1 and 4 h. Intervention shock dosing for a water quality problem (such as an accidental faecal release) may involve raising the free chlorine residual to 20 mg/l for an 8-h period while the pool is empty (see Section 5.8).
- Trying to compensate for inadequacies in treatment by shock dosing is bad practice, because it can mask deficiencies in design or operation that may produce other problems.
- If not enough chlorine is added, the combined chlorine (chloramines) problem may be exacerbated, and conjunctival irritation and obnoxious odours in the pool area may be raised to high levels. If too much chlorine is added, it may take a long time to drop to safe levels before bathing can be resumed. Chlorine levels should return to acceptable levels (i.e. <5 mg/l – see Section 4.4.1) before bathers are permitted in the pool.

5.4 Filtration

The primary function of filtration is to remove turbidity to achieve appropriate water clarity. Water clarity is a key factor in ensuring the safety of swimmers. Poor underwater visibility is a contributing factor to injuries (Chapter 2) and can seriously hamper recognition of swimmers in distress or a body lying on the bottom of the pool.

Disinfection will also be compromised by particulates. Particles can shield microorganisms from the action of disinfectants. Alternatively, the disinfectants may react with certain components of organic particles to form complexes that are less effective than the parent compounds, or the disinfectants may oxidize the organic material, thereby eliminating disinfection potential. Filtration is often the critical step for the removal of *Cryptosporidium* oocysts and *Giardia* cysts (see Section 3.3). Filtration is also effective against microbes, notably free-living amoebae, that harbour opportunistic bacteria such as *Legionella* and *Mycobacterium* species.

5.4.1 Filter types

There are a number of types of filter available, and the choice of filter will be based on several factors, including:

- the quality of the source water;
- the amount of filter area available and number of filters> Pools benefit greatly from the increased flexibility and safeguards of having more than one filter;

- filtration rate: Typically, the higher the filtration rate, the lower the filtration efficiency;
- ease of operation;
- method of backwashing: The cleaning of a filter bed clogged with solids is referred to as backwashing. It is accomplished by reversing the flow, fluidizing the filter material and passing pool water back through the filters to waste. Backwashing should be done as recommended by the filter manufacturer, when the allowable turbidity value has been exceeded, when a certain length of time without backwashing has passed or when a pressure differential is observed; and
- degree of operator training required.

1. Cartridge filters

Cartridge filters can nominally filter down to 7 μm and last up to two years. The filter medium is spun-bound polyester or treated paper. Cleaning is achieved by removing the cartridge and washing it. Their main advantage is the relatively small space requirement compared with other filter types, and they are often used with small pools and hot tubs.

2. Sand filters

Medium-rate sand filters can nominally filter down to about 7 μm in size with the addition of a suitable coagulant (such as polyaluminium chloride or aluminium hydroxychloride). Cleaning is achieved by manual reverse flow backwashing, with air scouring to remove body oils and fats to improve the backwash efficiency. For indoor heated pools, the sand medium typically has a life of between five and seven years. Medium-rate sand filters are comparatively large-diameter pressure vessels (in a horizontal or vertical format) and require large plant rooms. Drinking-water treatment has shown that when operated with a coagulant, sand filters can remove over 99% of *Cryptosporidium* oocysts. Studies in a pilot sand filtration plant under swimming pool filtration conditions have shown that without the addition of coagulant, removal of the *Cryptosporidium* oocyst surrogate (fluorescent polystyrene particles sized between 1 and 7 μm) was less than 50%. Using coagulants, polyaluminium chloride and polyaluminium silicate sulfate improved the removal up to 99% (Pool Water Treatment Advisory Group, pers. comm.).

3. Ultrafine filters

Ultrafine precoat filters (UFF) use a replaceable filter medium that is added after each backwash. Filter media include diatomaceous earth, diatomite products and perlite. The benefit of precoat filtration is that it can provide a particle removal of 1–2 μm and, as such, provide good removal of *Cryptosporidium* oocysts. Table 5.1 compares the alternative filter types.

5.4.2 Turbidity measurement

Turbidity is a measure of the amount of suspended matter in water, and the more turbid the water, the less clarity. Turbidity needs to be controlled both for safety and for effective disinfection. For identifying bodies at the bottom of the pool, a universal turbidity value is not considered to be appropriate, as much depends on the characteristics of the individual pool, such as surface reflection and pool material/construction. Individual standards should be developed, based on risk assessment at each pool,

Table 5.1. Comparison of filter types

Criteria	Filter type		
	UFF	Medium-rate sand	Cartridge
Common filter sizes	Up to 46 m²	Up to 10 m²	Up to 20 m²
Design filter flow rate	3–5 m³/m²/h	25–30 m³/m²/h	1.5 m³/m²/h
Cleaning flow rate	5 m³/m²/h	37–42 m³/m²/h	Not applicable
Cleaning	Backwash and media replacement	Backwash	Manual, hose down
Average wash water	0.25 m³/m² pool water	2.5 m³/m² pool water	0.02 m³/m² mains water
Filter aid	None	Optional coagulants	None
Cleaning implications	A backwash tank may be required. Separation tank required to collect used filter media with periodic sludge removal	A backwash tank may be required	Hose-down and waste drain facility
Particulate collection	Surface	Depth	Degree of depth
Nominal particle removal	1–2 μm	10 μm, 7 μm with coagulant	7 μm
Pressure rise for backwash	70 kPa	40 kPa	40 kPa
Comparative running costs	High	Low	Medium
Comparative installation costs	High	High	Low

UFF = ultrafine filter

but it is recommended that, as a minimum, it should be possible to see a small child at the bottom of the pool from the lifeguard position while the water surface is in movement, as in normal use. An alternative is to maintain water clarity so that lane markings or other features on the pool bottom at its greatest depth are clearly visible when viewed from the side of the pool. Operators could determine these indicators as a turbidity equivalent through experience and then monitor routinely for turbidity. In terms of effective disinfection, a useful, but not absolute, upper-limit guideline for turbidity is 0.5 nephelometric turbidity unit (NTU), determined by the nephelometric method (ISO, 1999).

5.5 Dilution

Coagulation, filtration and disinfection will not remove all pollutants. Swimming pool design should enable the dilution of pool water with fresh water. Dilution limits the build-up of pollutants from bathers (e.g. constituents of sweat and urine), of by-products of disinfection and of various other dissolved chemicals. Dilution rates need to account for the replacement of water used in filter backwashing, evaporation and splash-out. As a general rule, the addition of fresh water to disinfected pools should not be less than 30 litres per bather.

5.6 Circulation and hydraulics

The purpose of paying close attention to circulation and hydraulics is to ensure that the whole pool is adequately served by filtered, disinfected water. Treated water must get to all parts of the pool, and polluted water must be removed – especially from areas most used and most polluted by bathers. It is recommended that 75–80% be taken from the surface (where the pollution is greatest – Gansloser et al., 1999), with the remainder taken from the bottom of the pool. The bottom returns allow the removal of grit and improved circulation within the pool. Without good circulation and hydraulics, even water treatment may not give adequate pool water quality.

The circulation rate is defined as the flow of water to and from the pool through all the pipework and the treatment system. The appropriate circulation rate depends, in most cases, on bathing load. There are, however, some types of pool where circulation rate cannot realistically be derived from bathing load – diving pools and other waters more than 2 m deep, for example, where the bathing load relative to water volume may be very low. Circulation rate is related to turnover period, which is the time taken for a volume of water equivalent to the entire pool water volume to pass through the filters and treatment plant and back to the pool. Turnover periods must, however, also suit the particular type of pool (see Box 5.1 for an example of guidance); this is related to the likely pollution load based on the type of activity undertaken and the volume of water within the pool. Where pools have moveable floors, the turnover should be calculated based upon the shallowest depth achievable. Formulae are available for calculating turnover rates, and these should be employed at the design stage. Box 5.1 gives some examples of turnover periods that have been employed in the UK.

BOX 5.1 EXAMPLES OF TURNOVER PERIODS FOR DIFFERENT TYPES OF POOLS

In the United Kingdom (BSI, 2003), the following turnover periods for different types of pools have been recommended:

Pool type	Turnover period
Competition pools 50 m long	3–4 h
Conventional pools up to 25 m long with 1-m shallow end	2.5–3 h
Diving pools	4–8 h
Hydrotherapy pools	0.5–1 h
Leisure water bubble pools	5–20 min
Leisure waters up to 0.5 m deep	10–45 min
Leisure waters 0.5–1 m deep	0.5–1.25 h
Leisure waters 1–1.5 m deep	1–2 h
Leisure waters over 1.5 m deep	2–2.5 h
Teaching/learner/training pools	0.5–1.5 h
Water slide splash pools	0.5–1 h

5.7 Bathing load

Bathing load is a measure of the number of people in the pool. For a new pool, the bathing load should be estimated at the design stage.

There are many factors that determine the maximum bathing load for a pool; these include:

- area of water – in terms of space for bathers to move around in and physical safety;
- depth of water – the deeper the water, the more actual swimming there is and the more area a bather requires;

- comfort; and
- pool type and bathing activity.

Pool operators need to be aware of the maximum bathing load and should ensure that it is not exceeded during the operation of the pool. Where the maximum bathing load has not been established, it has been suggested in the UK that the figures in Table 5.2 (BSI, 2003) can provide an approximation. These figures may not be appropriate for all pool types or all countries.

Table 5.2. An example of maximum bathing loads[a]

Water depth	Maximum bathing load
<1.0 m	1 bather per 2.2 m^2
1.0–1.5 m	1 bather per 2.7 m^2
>1.5 m	1 bather per 4.0 m^2

[a] Adapted from BSI, 2003

5.8 Accidental release of faeces or vomit into pools

Accidental faecal releases may occur relatively frequently, although it is likely that most go undetected. Accidental faecal releases into swimming pools and similar environments can lead to outbreaks of infections associated with faecally-derived viruses, bacteria and pathogenic protozoa (Chapter 3); vomit may have a similar effect. A pool operator faced with an accidental faecal release or vomit in the pool water must, therefore, act immediately.

If the faecal release is a solid stool, it should simply be retrieved quickly and discarded appropriately. The scoop used to retrieve it should be disinfected so that any bacteria and viruses adhering to it are inactivated and will not be returned to the pool the next time the scoop is used. As long as the pool is, in other respects, operating properly (i.e. disinfectant levels are maintained), no further action is necessary. The same applies to solid animal faeces.

If the stool is runny (diarrhoea) or if there is vomit, the situation is more likely to be hazardous, as the faeces or vomit is more likely to contain pathogens. Even though most disinfectants deal relatively well with many bacterial and viral agents in accidental faecal releases and vomit, the possibility exists that the diarrhoea or vomit is from someone infected with one of the protozoan parasites, *Cryptosporidium* and *Giardia*. The infectious stages (oocysts/cysts) are resistant to chlorine disinfectants in the concentrations that are practical to use. The pool should therefore be cleared of bathers immediately.

The safest action, if the incident has occurred in a small pool or hot tub, is to empty and clean it before refilling and reopening. However, this is practically impossible in many larger pools, for reasons of cost and extended periods of closure. If draining down is not possible, then a procedure based on the one given below should be followed (it should be noted, however, that this is an imperfect solution that will only reduce but not eliminate risk):

- The pool should be cleared of people immediately.
- As much of the material as possible should be collected, removed and disposed of to waste; this may be done through netting, sweeping and/or vacuuming (provided the equipment can be adequately disinfected after use).

- Disinfectant levels should be maintained at the top of the recommended range *or* chlorination to 20 mg/l at pH 7.2–7.5 for 8 h (shock dosing) should be performed.
- Using a coagulant (if appropriate), the water should be filtered for six turnover cycles; this may mean closing the pool until the next day.
- The filter should be backwashed (and the water run to waste).
- The final residual disinfectant level and pH value should be checked, and if satisfactory, then the pool can be reopened.

The willingness of operators and lifeguards to act is critical. Pool operators are unlikely to know with certainty what has caused a diarrhoea incident, and a significant proportion of such diarrhoea incidents may happen without lifeguards being aware of them. The most important contribution a pool operator can make to the problem is to guard against it. There are a few practical actions pool operators can take to help prevent faecal release into pools:

- No child (or adult) with a recent history of diarrhoea should swim.
- Parents should be encouraged to make sure their children use the toilet before they swim, and babies and toddlers that have not been toilet trained should ideally wear waterproof nappies or specially designed bathing wear.
- Young children *should whenever possible* be confined to pools small enough to drain in the event of an accidental release of faeces or vomit.
- Lifeguards should be made responsible for looking out for and acting on accidental faecal release/vomit incidents.

5.9 Air quality

Air quality in indoor swimming pool facilities is important for a number of reasons, including:

- Staff and user health. The quantity of water treatment by-products, concentration of airborne particulate matter and fresh air need to be controlled. The two areas of principal concern for health are *Legionella* and disinfection by-products, particularly chloramines. Although *Legionella* should primarily be controlled in the water systems, areas housing natural spas (thermal water) and hot tubs should also be well ventilated. Reducing exposure to disinfection by-products in air should be pursued in order to minimize overall exposure to these chemicals, as inhalation appears to be the dominant route of exposure during recreational water use (see Chapter 4). As concentrations of disinfection by-products decrease rapidly with distance from the water, this has implications for ventilation design, which involves both mixing and dilution (i.e. with fresh air), and building codes should stipulate appropriate ventilation rates (at least 10 litres of fresh air/s/m^2 of water surface area).
- Staff and user comfort. The temperature, humidity and velocity of the pool hall air should be appropriate to provide a comfortable environment.
- Impact on the building fabric. The air temperature, concentration of airborne particulate matter and quantity of water treatment by-products need to be controlled in order to avoid an 'aggressive environment' that may damage the building fabric.

5.10 Monitoring

Parameters that are easy and inexpensive to measure reliably and of immediate operational health relevance (such as turbidity, residual disinfectant and pH) should be monitored most frequently and in all pool types. Whether any other parameters (physical, chemical and microbial) need to be monitored is, in practice, determined by management capacity, intensity of use and local practice. However, microbial monitoring is generally needed in public and semi-public pools.

There should be pre-established (clear, written) procedures set up by managers for acting on the results of monitoring, including how to act on any unexpected results. Operators must know what to do themselves or how to ensure that appropriate action is taken by someone else. Management should review data and test systems regularly and ensure that pool operators have taken appropriate remedial action.

5.10.1 Turbidity

Turbidity testing is simple; approaches to establishing appropriate, facility-specific turbidity standards are described in Section 5.4.2. Exceedance of a turbidity standard suggests both a significant deterioration in water quality and a significant health hazard. Such exceedance merits immediate investigation and should lead to facility closure unless the turbidity can rapidly be brought within standards.

5.10.2 Residual disinfectant level

National or other standards for minimum and maximum levels of residual disinfectant vary widely. The main factor is that the residual disinfectant level should always be consistent with satisfactory microbial quality.

Failure to maintain target residual disinfectant should result in immediate investigation and follow-up testing. If residuals cannot be rapidly re-established and maintained, then full investigation of cause and prevention of repetition are merited, and public health authorities should be consulted in determining whether the facility should remain open.

1. Chlorine-based disinfectants

For a conventional public or semi-public swimming pool with good hydraulics and filtration, operating within its design bathing load and turnover and providing frequent (or online) monitoring of chlorine and pH, experience has shown that adequate routine disinfection should be achieved with a free chlorine level of 1 mg/l throughout the pool. Free chlorine levels well above 1.2 mg/l should not be necessary anywhere in the pool unless the pool is not well designed or well operated – if, for example, circulation is too slow, distribution is poor or bathing loads are too heavy; where this is the case, it is more appropriate in the long term to deal with the underlying problem, rather than increasing disinfection levels.

Experience suggests that the combined chlorine level within pool water (chloramines) should be no more than half the free chlorine level (but combined chlorine should be as low as possible and ideally less than 0.2 mg/l). If the levels are high, then it is likely that there is too much ammonia in the water, indicating that bathing loads or pollution from bathers may be too high, that dilution is too low or that treatment is suboptimal.

Lower free chlorine concentrations (0.5 mg/l or less) will be adequate where chlorine is used in conjunction with ozone or UV disinfection. Higher concentrations (up to 2–3 mg/l) may be required to ensure disinfection in hot tubs, because of higher bathing loads and higher temperatures.

If the chlorine source is chlorinated isocyanurate compounds, then the level of cyanuric acid must also be monitored and controlled; if it becomes too high (above 100 mg/l), microbial conditions may become unsatisfactory, and increased freshwater dilution is required.

2. Bromine-based disinfectants

Total bromine levels in swimming pools, should ideally be maintained at 2.0–2.5 mg/l. When bromine-based disinfectants are used in combination with ozone, the concentration of bromide ion should be monitored and maintained at 15–20 mg/l. If BCDMH is the bromine source, the level of dimethylhydantoin must also be monitored; it should not exceed 200 mg/l.

3. Sampling and analysis

In public and many semi-public pools, there will be continuous monitoring of residual disinfectant levels as the disinfectant is dosed (see Section 5.3.4). In addition to this, samples should also be taken from the pool itself. In public and semi-public pools, residual disinfectant concentrations should be checked by sampling the pool before it opens and during the opening period (ideally during a period of high bathing load). The frequency of testing while the swimming pool is in use depends upon the nature and use of the pool. It is suggested that the residual disinfectant concentration in domestic pools be checked before use. All tests must be carried out immediately after the sample is taken.

Samples should be taken at a depth of 5–30 cm. It is good practice to include as a routine sampling point the area of the pool where, because of the hydraulics, the disinfectant residual is generally lowest. Occasional samples should be taken from other parts of the pool and circulation system.

The tests employed should be capable of determining free chlorine and total bromine levels (depending upon the disinfectant used). Analysis is generally performed with simple test kits based on the N,N-diethyl-p-phenylenediamine (DPD) method, using either liquid or tablet reagents. This method can measure both free and total disinfectant and is available as both colorimetric and titration test kits.

5.10.3 pH

The pH of swimming pool water should be controlled to ensure efficient disinfection and coagulation, to avoid damage to the pool fabric and ensure user comfort. The pH should be maintained between 7.2 and 7.8 for chlorine disinfectants and between 7.2 and 8.0 for bromine-based and other non-chlorine processes. The frequency of measurement will depend upon the type of pool. It is suggested that for public pools, the pH value should be measured continuously and adjusted automatically; for other semi-public pools and public and semi-public hot tubs, it is suggested that monitoring be conducted several times a day, during operating hours; for domestic pools, it is advisable to measure prior to pool use. Actions to be taken on failure to maintain pH within the target range are similar to those for disinfectant residual.

5.10.4 Oxidation–reduction potential (ORP)

The oxidation–reduction potential (also known as ORP or redox) can also be used in the operational monitoring of disinfection efficacy. In general terms for swimming pools and similar environments, levels in excess of 720 mV (measured using a silver/silver chloride electrode) or 680 mV (using a calomel electrode) suggest that the water is in good microbial condition, although it is suggested that appropriate values should be determined on a case-by-case basis.

5.10.5 Microbial quality

There is limited risk of significant microbial contamination and illness in a well managed pool with an adequate residual disinfectant concentration, a pH value maintained at an appropriate level, well operated filters and frequent monitoring of non-microbial parameters. Nevertheless, samples of pool water from public and semi-public pools should be monitored at appropriate intervals for microbial parameters. Such tests do not guarantee microbial safety but serve to provide information with which to judge the effectiveness of measures taken.

1. 'Indicator' organisms

As outlined in Chapter 3, monitoring for potential microbial hazards is generally done using 'indicator' microorganisms, rather than specific microbial hazards (see Box 3.1). Microorganisms used to assess the microbial quality of pools and similar environments include heterotrophic plate count (HPC), thermotolerant coliforms, *E. coli*, *Pseudomonas aeruginosa*, *Legionella* spp. and *Staphylococcus aureus*. Where operational guidelines are exceeded, pool operators should check turbidity, residual disinfectant levels and pH and then resample. When critical guidelines are exceeded, the pool should be closed while investigation and remediation are conducted.

HPC
The HPC (37 °C for 24 h) gives an indication of the overall bacterial population within the pool. This should be monitored in public and semi-public disinfected swimming pools. It is recommended that operational levels should be less than 200 cfu/ml.

Thermotolerant coliforms and *E. coli*
Thermotolerant coliforms and *E. coli* are indicators of faecal contamination. Either thermotolerant coliforms **or** *E. coli* should be measured in all public and semi-public pools, hot tubs and natural spas. Operational levels should be less than 1/100 ml.

Pseudomonas aeruginosa
Routine monitoring of *Pseudomonas aeruginosa* is recommended for public and semi-public hot tubs and natural spas. It is suggested for public and semi-public swimming pools when there is evidence of operational problems (such as failure of disinfection or problems relating to filters or water pipes), a deterioration in the quality of the pool water or known health problems. It is recommended that for continuously disinfected pools, operational levels should be <1/100 ml; where natural spas operate with no residual disinfectant, operational levels should be <10/100 ml.

If high counts are found (>100/100 ml), pool operators should check turbidity, disinfectant residuals and pH, resample, backwash thoroughly, wait one turnover and resample. If high levels of *P. aeruginosa* remain, the pool should be closed and a thorough cleaning and disinfection programme initiated. Hot tubs should be shut down, drained, cleaned and refilled.

Legionella spp.
Periodic testing for *Legionella* is useful, especially from hot tubs, in order to determine that filters are not being colonized, and it is recommended that operational levels should be <1/100 ml. Where this is exceeded, hot tubs should be shut down, drained, cleaned and refilled. Shock chlorination may be appropriate if it is suspected that filters have become colonized.

Staphylococcus aureus
The routine monitoring of *Staphylococcus aureus* is not recommended, although monitoring may be undertaken as part of a wider investigation into the quality of the water when health problems associated with the pool are suspected. Where samples are taken, levels should be less than 100/100 ml.

2. *Sampling*
Guidelines on routine sampling frequencies, along with a summary of operational guideline values, are outlined in Table 5.3. In addition to routine sampling, samples should also be taken from public and semi-public facilities:

- before a pool is used for the first time;
- before it is put back into use, after it has been shut down for repairs or cleaning;
- if there are difficulties with the treatment system; and
- as part of any investigation into possible adverse effects on bathers' health.

Table 5.3. Recommended routine sampling frequencies[a] and operational guidelines[b] for microbial testing during normal operation

Pool type	Heterotrophic plate count	Thermotolerant coliform/*E. coli*	*Pseudomonas aeruginosa*	*Legionella* spp.
Disinfected pools, public and heavily used	Weekly (<200/ml)	Weekly (<1/100 ml)	When situation demands[c] (<1/100 ml)	Quarterly (<1/100 ml)
Disinfected pools, semi-public	Monthly (<200/ml)	Monthly (<1/100 ml)	When situation demands[c] (<1/100 ml)	Quarterly (<1/100 ml)
Natural spas	n/a	Weekly (<1/100 ml)	Weekly (<10/100 ml)	Monthly (<1/100 ml)
Hot tubs	n/a	Weekly (<1/100 ml)	Weekly (<1/100 ml)	Monthly (<1/100 ml)

[a] Samples should be taken when the pool is heavily loaded
Sampling frequency should be increased if operational parameters (e.g. turbidity, pH, residual disinfectant concentration) are not maintained within target ranges
Sample numbers should be determined on the basis of pool size and complexity and should include point(s) representative of general water quality and likely problem areas

[b] Operational guidelines are shown in parentheses

[c] e.g. when health problems associated with the pool are suspected

The most appropriate site for taking a single sample is where the water velocity is low, away from any inlets. Depending on the size of the pool, it may be advisable to take samples from multiple sites. Many leisure pools will have additional features, such as flumes, islands and backwaters with a complex system of water flow; representative samples should be taken.

Misleading information on pool water quality will result from incorrect sampling procedures. Sample containers must be of a material that will not affect the quality of the sample either microbially or chemically. Although a good-quality glass container will meet these requirements, the risk of broken glass in the pool environment as a result of breakage has favoured the use of shatterproof plastic-coated glass containers. All-plastic containers can be used provided they do not react with microorganisms or chemicals in the water; not all are suitable.

For microbial examination, the bottle must be sterile and contain an agent that neutralizes the disinfectant used in the pool water. Sodium thiosulfate (18–20 mg/l) is the agent used for chlorine- and bromine-based disinfectants. Clearly, the testing laboratory must be advised before sampling if any other disinfectant is being used. Bacteria in pool water samples and especially those from disinfected pools may be 'injured', and normal analytical 'resuscitation' procedures should be fully adhered to.

5.10.6 *Other operational parameters*

Several parameters are important for operational purposes. These include:

- *alkalinity*: Alkalinity is a measure of the alkaline salts dissolved in the water. The higher the alkalinity, the more resistant the water is to large changes in pH in response to changes in the dosage of disinfectant and pH correction chemicals. If the alkalinity is too high, it can make pH adjustment difficult.
- *calcium hardness*: Calcium hardness is an operational measure that needs to be monitored to avoid damage to the pool fabric (e.g. etching of surfaces and metal corrosion) and scaling water.
- *total dissolved solids*: Total dissolved solids (TDS) is the weight of soluble material in water. Disinfectants and other pool chemicals as well as bather pollution will increase TDS levels. The real value of detecting an increase in TDS levels is as a warning of overloading or lack of dilution, and TDS levels should be monitored by comparison between pool and source water. If TDS is high, dilution is likely to be the correct management action.

5.11 Cleaning

Good water and air quality cannot be maintained without an adequate cleaning programme. This should include the toilets, showers, changing facilities and pool surroundings on at least a daily basis in public and semi-public pools. Public and semi-public hot tubs should be drained and the surfaces and pipework cleaned on a weekly basis. Heating, ventilation and air-conditioning systems should be cleaned periodically (e.g. weekly to monthly for those serving hot tubs). Features such as water sprays should be periodically cleaned and flushed with disinfectant (e.g. 5 mg/l hypochlorite solution).

5.12 References

BSI (2003) *Management of public swimming pools – water treatment systems, water treatment plant and heating and ventilation systems – code of practice.* British Standards Institute, Publicly Available Specification (PAS) 39: 2003.

Eichelsdörfer D (1987) [Investigations of anthropogenic load of swimming pool and bathing water.] *A.B. Archiv des Badewesens*, 40: 259–263 (in German).

Eichelsdörfer D, Jandik J (1979) [Ozone as oxidizer.] *A.B. Archiv des Badewesens*, 37: 257–261 (in German).

Eichelsdörfer D, Jandik J (1984) [Investigation and development of swimming pool water treatment. III. Note: Pool water treatment with ozone in long time contact.] *Zeitschrift für Wasser- und Abwasser Forschung*, 17: 148–153 (in German).

Eichelsdörfer D, Jandik J, Weil

(1981) [Formation and occurrence of organic halocarbons in swimming pool water.] *A.B. Archiv des Badewesens*, 34: 167–172 (in German).

Gansloser G, Hässelbarth U, Roeske W (1999) [*Treatment of swimming pool and bathing water.*] Berlin, Beuth Verlag (in German).

Gregory R (2002) Bench-marking pool water treatment for coping with *Cryptosporidium. Journal of Environmental Health Research*, 1(1): 11–18.

ISO (1999) *Water quality – Determination of turbidity.* Geneva, International Organization for Standardization (ISO 7027:1999).

Locher A (1996) [Non-chlorine treatment of pool water.] *Gesundheits- und Umwelttechnik*, 3: 18–19 (in German).

MDHSS (undated) *Swimming pool and spa water chemistry.* Missouri Department of Health and Senior Services, Section for Environmental Health (http://www.health.state.mo.us/RecreationalWater/Pool SpaChem.pdf).

Rice RG (1995) Chemistries of ozone for municipal pool and spa water treatment. *Journal of the Swimming Pool and Spa Industry*, 1(1): 25–44.

Saunus C (1998) [*Planning of swimming pools.*] Düsseldorf, Krammer Verlag (in German).

CHAPTER 6
Guideline implementation

Recreational water activities can bring health benefits to users, including exercise and relaxation. However, negative health effects may also arise as described in previous chapters. It is necessary to address these issues and implement effective management options in order to minimize the adverse health consequences through implementation of the Guidelines.

Different stakeholders play different roles in the management of the recreational water environment for safety. The typical areas of responsibility may be grouped into four major categories, although there may be overlap between these and stakeholders with responsibilities falling within more than one category:

- design and construction;
- operation and management;
- public education and information; and
- regulatory requirements (including compliance).

This chapter is arranged according to these categories, with the main stakeholders indicated for each category. Successful implementation of the Guidelines will require development of suitable capacities and expertise and the elaboration of a coherent policy and legislative framework.

6.1 Design and construction

People responsible for commissioning pools and similar environments, along with designers and contractors, should be aware of the requirements to ensure safe and enjoyable use of facilities. Many decisions taken at the design and construction stage will have repercussions on the ease with which safe operation can be ensured once the pool is in use.

Table 6.1 summarizes examples of good practice in design, specification or construction of swimming pools and similar environments in relation to the major health issues discussed in previous chapters, while Table 6.2 examines specific risks in various pool types in relation to design and construction issues.

Local and national authorities may set specific requirements that must be met in the design and construction of swimming pools and similar recreational water facilities (see also Section 6.4). Alternatively, less formal guidelines may be established by these authorities or by professional or trade associations. Competent and experienced persons may be members of professional associations or may be subject to licensing schemes in order to practise (see Section 6.4.2). There may be a process of approval for design and during construction – for example, through building regulations.

Table 6.1. Examples of good practice in design and construction: major health-related issues

Objective[a]	Typical actions/requirements of good practice
Prevention of entrapment injuries (2)	Specify minimum two suction drains per pump system, with drains sufficiently separated to prevent trapping. Properly installed outlets and drain grates to prevent suction entrapment. Pump shut-off permanently accessible to lifeguards or public (if no permanent lifeguard).
Prevention of diving accidents (2)	Clear indication of depth in locally comprehensible manner at frequent intervals.
Enable adequate lifeguarding (2)	All areas of pool visible from lifeguarding posts. Adequate artificial light. Glare does not impede underwater visibility. Plain pool bottom assists recognition of bodies.
Prevention of slip/trip/fall accidents (2)	Non-slip surround surfaces. Area bordering pool clear of tripping hazards (e.g. pipes and equipment). Temporary fixtures create no hazard when removed (e.g. starting blocks). Pool surround sloped to drain effectively. Edge of pool surround in contrasting colour (unless gentle slope from surface). Steps, treads, etc. marked by contrasting colour. Pool and surround free of sharp edges or projections.
Minimize unintentional immersion and enable self-recovery (especially for non-swimmers) (2)	Avoid unauthorized access, isolation fencing (enclosing the pool only) at least 1.2 m high with self-closing, self-latching gate is recommended for pools where children could obtain unsupervised access. Avoid abrupt changes in depth, especially in shallow (e.g. <1.5 m depth) waters. Changes in depth identified by use of colour-contrasted materials. Side and end walls vertical for a minimum of 1 m. Steps/ladders for easy access in and out of pool.
Minimize and control faecal and non-faecal microbial contamination (3)	Provide easy access to toilets and showers. Design pre-swim showers so bathers have to shower before entrance to the pool area. Strategic placement of footbaths. Provision of adequate treatment capacity. On commissioning or after equipment change or modification to pipes, drains, etc., confirm circulation pattern and absence of 'dead spots' (e.g. by dye tests). For public and semi-public pools (where possible), include small, separate pools for children to facilitate draining in response to accidental faecal releases.
Minimize exposure to volatile chemicals (4)	Ensure air flow across water surface (forced or natural ventilation) and adequate fresh air exchange.
Minimize formation of disinfection by-products by control of precursor input (5)	Design pool treatment system to reduce DBP formation (e.g. water pre-treatment if necessary, disinfection systems that use less chlorine – e.g. UV or ozone plus chlorine). Provide easy-access toilets and showers.

[a] Relevant chapter references are identified in parentheses

Table 6.2. Health risks and design and construction issues associated with various pool types

Pool type or use (refer to Chapter 1)	Special risk factors[a]	Principal requirement/action
Natural spa waters (coloured or turbid)	Inability of users to see changes of depth (2) Inability of lifeguards to see bodies under surface (2)	No sudden underwater depth changes or steps
Flow-through seawater swimming pools on cruise ships and ferries	Polluted water in harbour areas Injuries during ship movement in heavy seas	Refer to WHO *Guide to Ship Sanitation* (in preparation)
Open-air pools	Unauthorized access to children (2) (e.g. when the pool is closed or unsupervised)	Exclusion of unsupervised children through fencing, walls with child-proof gates/doors
	Algal growth (5)	Best controlled by good hydraulic design
	Contamination by mud and grass on users' feet (5)	Provision of pre-swim showers and footbaths
	Contamination by animal faeces, animal urine and wind-blown matter (3 and 5)	Exclusion of animals Edge drainage draining away from the pool Ensuring adequate treatment capacity and good circulation and hydraulic design
Semi-public pools	Lack of adequate water quality management increases the risk of illness (3)	Water quality best controlled by ensuring appropriate treatment capacity, the inclusion of automatic monitoring and chemical dosing systems and good circulation and hydraulic design
Domestic pools (including temporary and portable pools)	Unauthorized access to children (2) (i.e. when the pool is unsupervised)	Provision of isolation fencing with child-proof gates
Hot tubs	Unauthorized access to children (2) (i.e. when the hot tub is unsupervised)	Provision of lockable safety covers on domestic and outdoor hot tubs
	Difficulty in maintaining an appropriate residual disinfectant level (3 and 4)	Provide identifiable seats to prevent overcrowding. Facility designed to enable 'rest periods' to be programmed, to discourage excessive use and allow disinfectant levels to 'recover'
	Temperature too hot	Pre-set maximum temperature <40 °C

[a] Relevant chapter references are identified in parentheses

Equipment specified or purchased should meet prevailing standards (see Section 6.4.2). In addition, guidance may be available with regards to the most suitable materials to use for construction to minimize problems with corrosion.

6.2 Operation and management

Facility operators play a key role and are responsible for the good operation and management of the recreational water environment. Good operation is vital to minimize possible negative health impacts. Table 6.3 summarizes examples of good practice in operation and management to deal with the hazards identified in previous chapters.

Table 6.4 examines specific risks in relation to good operation and management by pool type.

6.2.1 Pool safety plan

The facility operator should have a pool safety plan, which consists of a description of the system, its monitoring and maintenance, normal operating procedures, a set of procedures for specified incidents, an emergency evacuation procedure and a generic emergency plan (for things not covered under the specified incidents). Examples of what should be included within the normal operating procedure are outlined in Box 6.1.

BOX 6.1 EXAMPLES OF NORMAL OPERATING PROCEDURES

1. Details of the pool(s); this should include dimensions and depths, features and equipment and a plan of the whole facility. The plan should include positions of pool alarms, fire alarms, emergency exit routes and any other relevant information.
2. Potential risk; a description of the main hazards and user groups particularly at risk is required before safe operating procedures can be identified.
3. Dealing with the public; arrangements for communicating safety messages to customers, ensuring maximum bather numbers are not exceeded, customer care and poolside rules.
4. Lifeguard's duties and responsibilities (see Section 6.2.2), including special supervision requirements for equipment, etc., lifeguard training and numbers of lifeguards for particular activities.
5. Systems of work, including lines of supervision, call-out procedures, work rotation and maximum poolside working times.
6. Controlling access to a pool or pools intended to be out of use, including the safe use of pool covers.
7. Water quality monitoring, including how often, how and where samples are to be taken, details of the operational and critical limits and actions to be taken if water quality is not satisfactory.
8. Response to an accidental faecal release (or this may be covered under an incident plan).
9. Detailed work instructions, including pool cleaning procedures, safe setting up and checking of equipment and setting up the pool for galas.
10. First-aid supplies and training, including equipment required, its location, arrangements for checking it, first aiders, first-aid training and disposal of sharp objects.
11. Details of alarm systems and any emergency equipment, maintenance arrangements; all alarm systems and emergency equipment provided, including operation, location, action to be taken on hearing the alarm, testing arrangements and maintenance.
12. Conditions of hire to, or use by, outside organizations.

Adapted from Sport England & Health and Safety Commission, 2003

Table 6.3. Good practice in operation and management: major health-related issues

Objective[a]	Typical actions/requirements of good practice
Prevention of drowning incidents (2)	Provision of properly trained and equipped lifeguards. Declared procedure for dealing with emergencies, all staff trained and familiar. Water turbidity monitored and action plan in place to deal with trends or deviations from acceptable range. Natural spas and hot tubs operated at temperatures below 40 °C. Ensuring unauthorized access is prevented. Installation and maintenance of appropriate water safety signage.[b] Forbidding consumption or sale of alcohol at recreational facility.
Prevention of diving injuries (2)	Signage[b] against diving into shallower water, active lifeguard supervision and intervention supported by management. Starting blocks and diving boards inaccessible to untrained persons. High boards with non-slip surfaces and side rails. Where possible (larger pools), designated areas for non-swimmers and children, increased supervision.
Prevention of entrapment injuries (2)	Checking that drain covers are in place and undamaged. Emergency shut-off is clearly marked.
Prevention of slip/trip/fall accidents (2)	Regular cleaning programme for all surfaces subject to algal or bacterial growth. Minimize presence of moveable objects (i.e. objects that could be transported near to pool edge and constitute a trip hazard).
Accident response capability (2)	Written emergency evacuation procedure and generic emergency plan. Rescue and resuscitation equipment available to lifeguards. First-aid equipment readily available. Communication links to local emergency and first-aid facilities readily available.
Control after accidental faecal releases (3 and 5)	Declared procedure for dealing with accidental faecal releases, all staff trained and familiar. For example: • Evacuation of pool immediately after accidental faecal releases. • Pool maintained out of use for a specified period, six full turnovers of filtration cycle during which disinfectant concentrations to be elevated and maintained at maximum normal operating concentration. • Total drain-down and cleaning of children's pools.
Maintenance of water quality and clean ancillary facilities (3 and 5)	Encouraging users to shower before using the facilities (e.g. through the use of posters and educational material – see also Section 6.3). Stated water quality and facilities monitoring programme implemented and recorded by trained staff. Respect bathing load limits. Declared process for dealing with adverse trends and unacceptable values. Previous identification of source of expertise/reference in case of problems. Availability of critical parameter water-testing equipment. Filtration performance periodically monitored and action taken if outside operational requirements. Maintenance of toilets, showers and changing rooms in clean, socially acceptable state.
Maintenance of air quality (5)	Manage DBP formation by encouraging users to shower before using the facilities. Monitoring. Ensuring adequate ventilation, especially across the pool surface, and suitable exchange with fresh air.

[a] Chapter references are given in parentheses
[b] Signage is also an education issue and is covered in more detail in Section 6.3.1

The normal operating procedures cover day-to-day management and aim to prevent problems such as poor air and water quality or overcrowding from arising, through monitoring and appropriate management actions. In terms of water quality monitoring, for a number of parameters there will be both operational and critical limits (see Section 5.10). When operational limits are exceeded, action should be taken to bring levels back in line with guidelines or standards. When a critical limit is exceeded, more urgent action is required, which may include closing the facility.

In addition to normal operating procedures, it is also necessary to have a series of incident plans that cover less routine matters, such as an accident to a water slide user (see Box 6.2) or how to manage an accidental faecal release (if this is not covered under the normal operating procedure – see Section 5.8).

Situations that are not covered by either the normal operating procedure or the incident plans are likely to be unanticipated emergency situations such as structural failure and should be dealt with according to an emergency evacuation procedure. The pool safety plan should be fully documented and the results of monitoring and any incidents recorded.

6.2.2 Lifeguards
The primary responsibilities of the lifeguard include the following (Sport England & Health and Safety Commission, 2003):

- supervising the pool area, keeping a close watch over the pool and its users;
- preventing injuries by minimizing or eliminating hazardous situations, intervening to prevent unsafe behaviours, exercising appropriate control and enforcing all facility rules and regulations;
- anticipating problems and preventing accidents, including warning bathers of the risks of their specific behaviours;
- identifying emergencies quickly and responding effectively, including effecting a rescue from the water, administering first aid or CPR, and informing other lifeguards and facility staff when more help or equipment is needed; and
- communicating with the pool users and colleagues.

Secondary responsibilities should not interfere with the primary responsibilities of lifeguard personnel. These secondary responsibilities include informing patrons about rules and regulations, helping patrons locate a missing person, completing required records and reports on schedule and submitting them to the proper person or office, and undertaking maintenance or other tasks as assigned.

A detailed example of the duties and requirements of a lifeguard and determination of lifeguard staffing levels are outlined in Appendix 1.

6.3 Public education and information
Facility operators, local authorities, public health bodies, pool-based clubs (such as swimming clubs, aqua-aerobics classes, scuba clubs and so on) and sports bodies can play an important role in ensuring pool safety through public education and providing appropriate and targeted information to pool users. Table 6.5 outlines education requirements and responses to identified risks by pool type.

Table 6.4. Health risks and operation and management actions associated with various pool types

Pool type or use (refer to Chapter 1)	Special risk factors[a]	Principal requirement/action
Natural spa and thermal waters	High water temperatures (2) Microbial water quality if water is untreatable (problems may be encountered with filtration and/or disinfection) (3)	Limit temperatures to below 40 °C. Drain-down obligatory after accidental faecal release. Monitoring for faecal indicators required. Special water quality management regime typically requires, for example, physical cleaning of surfaces above and below water. Regular drain-down and a high rate of dilution to waste.
Flumes, wave machines, etc.	Increased accident hazards, inhibition of visibility (2)	More intensive supervision. Avoid overcrowding Pre-warning of change in water conditions.
Flow-through seawater swimming pools on cruise ships and ferries	Risk of contamination from sewage discharge in source water Injuries during ship movement in high seas	Refer to WHO *Guide to Ship Sanitation* (in preparation)
Open-air pools	Unauthorized access to children (2) (e.g. when the pool is closed or unsupervised)	Maintenance of fencing, walls with child-proof gates/doors.
	Exposure to UV radiation degrades residual disinfectant (5)	Close monitoring of residual disinfectant or use of stabilizer (e.g. chlorinated isocyanurates) to lessen degradation.
	Algal growth (5)	Ensuring effective disinfection and good hydraulic design. If problems persist, then proprietary algicides for swimming pool application may be used.
	Contamination by mud and grass on users' feet (5)	Encouragement of the use of pre-swim showers and footbaths. Cleaning and maintenance around the pool area.
	Contamination by animal faeces, animal urine and wind-blown matter (3 and 5)	Banning of pets. Removal of litter to discourage presence of animals. Cleaning. Ensuring effective disinfection and filtration as well as good water circulation.
Public and semi-public pools with access to alcohol	Increased inappropriate behaviour, reduced ability to cope, impaired judgement (2)	Recommendations that facilities are not used while under the influence of alcohol. Supervision required. Physical exclusion of access at unsupervised times.

Table 6.4. *(continued)*

Pool type or use (refer to Chapter 1)	Special risk factors[a]	Principal requirement/action
Domestic pools (including temporary and portable pools)	Unauthorized access to children (2) (e.g. when the pool is unsupervised)	Maintenance of isolation fencing with child-proof gates.
	Deterioration in water quality (3)	Monitor water quality. Drain pool (if small), wash and refill after an accidental faecal release.
Hot tubs	Unauthorized access to children (2) (e.g. when the hot tub is unsupervised)	Securing of safety covers on domestic and outdoor tubs.
	Aerosolization (3)	Limit temperature to below 40 °C. *Legionella*-specific management (see Section 3.4.1).
	Difficulties in maintaining disinfectant residual (5)	Increased disinfectant monitoring. Implementation of 'rest periods' during use to allow disinfectant levels to 'recover'.

[a] Relevant chapter references are identified in parentheses

---

BOX 6.2 EXAMPLE INCIDENT PLAN FOR LIFEGUARDS MONITORING A WAVE POOL OR WATER SLIDE

When you spot a user who needs help, follow this procedure:

- By immediately blowing one long, loud whistle blast, you notify your safety team that there is an incident. Once you have given the signal, members of the safety team can react to the situation.

- Stop the waves or slide dispatch. At a wave pool, hit the emergency stop button to be sure the waves are turned off. If you are on duty at the top of an attraction, do not dispatch any more riders. Communication between the top and bottom positions is vital.

- Determine which method of rescue is needed. If it is necessary to enter the water to make a rescue, use the entry most appropriate for the location you are lifeguarding. For example, you might use a compact jump from a head wall. If it isn't necessary to enter the water, use the appropriate equipment to help the victim.

- If you are not the lifeguard making the rescue, make sure the rescuing lifeguard's observation zone is covered.

- Once the situation is under control, the lifeguard who made the rescue completes and files an incident report as soon as time permits. This report form should have a diagram of the pool or activity on the back so that the location of the incident can be marked for future study.

- All equipment used in the rescue must be checked to ensure it remains in good condition and is returned to the appropriate location. Lifeguards return to duty, if able, and users are allowed to participate in the activity again if there are enough guards to cover it.

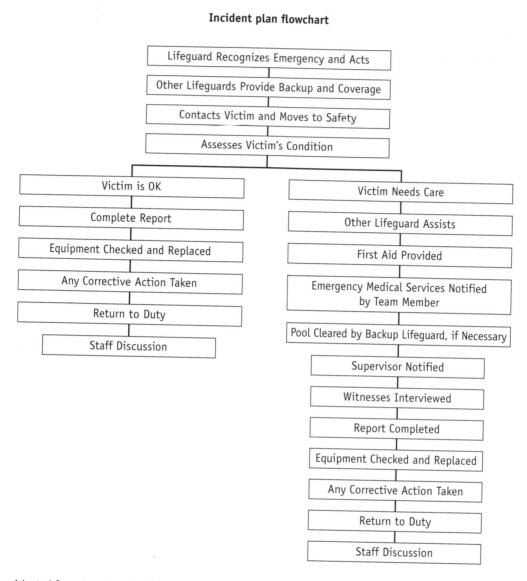

Incident plan flowchart

Lifeguard Recognizes Emergency and Acts

Other Lifeguards Provide Backup and Coverage

Contacts Victim and Moves to Safety

Assesses Victim's Condition

Victim is OK	Victim Needs Care
Complete Report	Other Lifeguard Assists
Equipment Checked and Replaced	First Aid Provided
Any Corrective Action Taken	Emergency Medical Services Notified by Team Member
Return to Duty	Pool Cleared by Backup Lifeguard, if Necessary
Staff Discussion	Supervisor Notified
	Witnesses Interviewed
	Report Completed
	Equipment Checked and Replaced
	Any Corrective Action Taken
	Return to Duty
	Staff Discussion

Adapted from American Red Cross, 1995

6.3.1 *Signage*

Information can be conveyed by means of prominently and appropriately located signs. These should provide concise information and a single message (as distinct from notices and posters, which are covered under Section 6.3.2). Signs can be used to inform people of hazards and safe behaviours and also reinforce previous educational messages. Warning signs, in particular, should be simple to understand and display a clear message. Many national organizations have adopted descriptive standards for warning and information signs, and the International Organization for

Table 6.5. Education to reduce health risks from special risk factors

Pool type or use (refer to Chapter 1)	Special risk factors[a]	Management action
Natural spa waters	Microbial water quality if water is untreatable (3)	Education for high-risk users on infection risk
Open-air pools	Unauthorized access to children (2) (e.g. when pool is unsupervised or closed)	Education of children and parents/caregivers on the drowning hazard posed by pools
	Water and air quality (5)	Education on the importance of pre-swim hygiene
Public and semi-public pools with access to alcohol	Increased inappropriate behaviour, reduced ability to cope, impaired judgement (2)	Information regarding peer supervision and safe behaviours, impact of alcohol
Domestic pools (including temporary and portable pools)	Unauthorized access to children (2)	Education of children and parents/caregivers on the drowning hazard posed by pools and hot tubs
Hot tubs	Aerosolization (3)	Education for high-risk users (such as young, elderly, pregnant women and immunocompromised) on infection risk and importance of avoiding excessive use
	Difficulties in maintaining residual disinfectant (5)	
	Overheating (2)	Alcohol warnings

[a] Relevant chapter references are identified in parentheses

Standardization (ISO) has adopted a standard for safety signs (not specifically swimming pool related) to try to avoid a proliferation of symbols that could cause confusion rather than send a clear message (ISO, 2003).

Signage can convey the need for awareness (e.g. danger), the hazard (e.g. shallow water), the health risk (e.g. paralysis may occur) or the prohibition (e.g. no diving, no running, no glass, no alcohol). Signage also includes pool labels and markings, such as pool depth markings. Extra attention may be required when designing signs applicable to tourist groups with different languages and cultures, as, unsurprisingly, some signs have been ineffective when such explanatory and precautionary information was in a language not understood by the pool users.

Signs alone may have a limited impact on behaviour (Hill, 1984; Goldhaber & de Turck, 1988). However, studies have shown that the public accept and recognize warning placards, pictographs and labelling. Therefore, signs are best deployed to reinforce previous awareness raising and education.

6.3.2 Education

Education can encourage pool, hot tub and natural spa users to adopt safer behaviours that benefit both themselves and other users and should encompass issues such as pre-swim hygiene, when not to use a pool or similar environment and how to identify possible hazards. Schools, public health bodies (including health care providers), facility operators and user groups can all provide information. Castor & Beach (2004), for example, suggest that health care providers can help to disseminate healthy swimming messages to their patients, especially those patients with diarrhoea and parents of children who are not toilet trained, or patients who are particularly susceptible to certain diseases or conditions. This would include messages on not swimming when you are suffering from diarrhoea, on showering before swimming or that immunocompromised patients should take extra precautions or not swim in areas with a higher probability of being contaminated.

Bather safety may be improved if possible hazards are clearly identified at the facility (see Section 6.3.1) and users educated before they enter the pool environment. An attempt at education may also be made by handing safety leaflets to users at the pool entrance or to those in charge of organized group activities and displaying posters in reception and changing room areas (Sport England & Health and Safety Commission, 2003). Lifeguards can also act as information providers, although this role should not interfere with their supervisory role.

Box 6.3 provides a code for pool users, which could be displayed in public areas or, where membership to a facility is required, form part of a membership pack. Educational information can also be added to agreements or contracts with groups that use pools for special purposes (e.g. scuba lessons, water aerobics, etc.).

BOX 6.3 EXAMPLE CODE FOR POOL USERS

Spot the dangers. Take care, swimming pools can be hazardous. Water presents a risk of drowning, and injuries can occur from hitting the hard surrounds or from misuse of the equipment. Every pool is different, so always make sure you know how deep the water is and check for other hazards, such as diving boards, wave machines, water slides, steep slopes into deeper water, etc.

Always swim within your ability. Never swim under the influence of alcohol. Avoid holding your breath and swimming long distances under water. Be especially careful if you have a medical condition such as epilepsy, asthma, diabetes or a heart problem. Follow advice provided for the safety of yourself and others. Avoid unruly behaviour that can be dangerous, for instance, running on the side of the pool, ducking, acrobatics in the water, or shouting or screaming (which could distract attention from an emergency). Always do as the lifeguards say, and remember that a moment of foolish behaviour could cost a life.

Look out for yourself and other swimmers. It is safer to swim with a companion. Keep an eye open for others, particularly younger children and non-swimmers. Learn how to help. If you see somebody in difficulty, call for help immediately. In an emergency, keep calm and do exactly as you are told.

Do not swim if you have a gastrointestinal (stomach) upset or skin or respiratory infection. You are likely to pass on the germs that are making you ill.

Shower before you swim. This will reduce the amount of germs, sweat and chemicals (such as cosmetics) that you transfer to the water. This means that the water quality of the pool will be better.

Adapted from Sport England & Health and Safety Commission, 2003

6.4 Regulatory requirements

National legislation may include different sets of regulations that will apply to swimming pools and similar recreational environments. Regulation may control, for example, the design and construction of pools (see Section 6.1), their operation and management (see

Section 6.2) and substances hazardous to health (e.g. chemicals). These may be quite detailed and specific in their requirements, covering water treatment processes, sampling and testing regimes, and they may be applied differently according to the type of pool (i.e. public versus semi-public versus domestic). Within regulations it is likely that there will be a requirement for the use of certified material, equipment and, possibly, staff registered to certain bodies (e.g. lifeguards, design and construction engineers).

Another aspect of pool management that may necessitate regulatory involvement is occupational health and safety legislation, designed to ensure protection of pool employees (occupational health is not covered by these Guidelines; see Chapter 1), as well as the general public.

Local regulatory oversight can support the work of pool management and provide greater public health protection and public confidence. Inspections by the regulatory officials to verify compliance with the regulations are an important component of this oversight.

6.4.1 Regulations and compliance

The extent to which swimming pools and similar environments are regulated varies greatly. In some countries, a permit or licence to operate is required by the local municipal authority. In others, a level of regulatory oversight is provided, based on specific regulations and/or advisory codes of practice.

Local authorities may, for example, require that the initial plans for the construction of a new pool be submitted by a licensed engineer. The design and construction plans are then reviewed and approved by a competent person. These plans generally include complete details and layout of the facility, including amenities, and information regarding the individual circulation system components (pumps, filters, chemical dosing system, etc.). Once approved, the construction of the facility may commence. However, prior to issuance of the final permit for operation, a physical inspection of the final facility and a review of the pool safety plan or daily operations management are usually required. Periodic audits may be required to ensure continued compliance. Regulations should provide for authority to close the facility if serious hazards and breaches to regulations or a significant risk to public health is identified, with reopening prohibited until the problem has been rectified and measures are in place to prevent recurrence.

Most regulations apply to public pools, but limited evidence suggests that the greatest burden of disease and physical injury arises from domestic and semi-public pools. These may be subject to periodic or informal supervision, and their operation and maintenance may be less adequate than those at public pools *per se*.

In terms of the operation and management of pools and similar environments, the typical requirements, in terms of a normal operating procedure, incident plans and an emergency plan, have already been outlined (Section 6.2). The preparation and use of such procedures ensure that the hazards specific to that facility have been evaluated and management actions determined.

It may be a regulatory requirement that the results of hygiene and safety monitoring be made available to the public; this may be useful in terms of public education material and, if the regulator also provides comparable information from other venues, as a means of comparing the health and safety records of different facilities.

In all cases, regulatory involvement should be welcomed and not seen as a burden on pool management. The purpose of regulatory involvement is to ensure that pools and similar environments are operated as safely as possible in order that the largest possible population gets the maximum possible benefit, not to close facilities or hinder their proper operation.

6.4.2 *Registration and certification schemes*

Certain staff members (e.g. lifeguards) and personnel involved in the design and construction (for example) may be required to be registered with certain approved bodies. In addition, all equipment components installed in the facility should meet minimum performance, design, sanitation and safety requirements. Certification that the equipment or the entire pool is in compliance with the guidelines or regulatory requirements is helpful for all involved parties. There are four basic methods of certification in use; these are outlined in Box 6.4.

Equipment that may be certified for performance, sanitation and/or safety considerations includes the following: piping system; filters; pumps; surface skimmers; suction fittings and drain covers; valves (multiport, three-way, butterfly, etc.); chemical feeding devices (mechanical, flow-through); process equipment (chlorine/bromine generators, ozone generators, UV disinfection systems and copper/silver ion generators); heaters; automated chemical monitor/controllers; chemical disinfectants; and electrical equipment (safety).

BOX 6.4 BASIC METHODS OF CERTIFICATION

- *First party* – Self-certification of the product's compliance against a standard by the manufacturer. Concerns are often raised with manufacturers' self-certification because of the potential bias of the manufacturer and the lack of ongoing monitoring to ensure that the product continues to comply.

- *Second party* – Certification by a trade association or private party. In many instances, trade associations or private companies provide testing and certification services for products against industry standards or regulations. Since a trade association represents and is often controlled by manufacturers, second-party certifications are not considered to be completely independent. Typically, no follow-up services to monitor continued compliance are provided. As a result, it is often difficult to determine whether a product selected for use is identical to the unit that was originally evaluated for certification. Private entities also offer testing and certification services that monitor the continued compliance of the product. These follow-up services often include audits of the production location, ongoing testing and complaint investigation.

- *Third party* – Certification by an independent organization without direct ties to the manufacturing sector. Third-party certifications provide for an independent evaluation of the product coupled with follow-up services that help ensure that products continue to comply with all requirements. These follow-up services typically include audits of the production location, ongoing testing of representative products and complaint investigation. The follow-up service aspect of third-party certification is an advantage, in that the purchaser has the assurance that the product installed is identical to the product evaluated for the certification. Third-party certifiers also maintain close working relationships with the regulatory and user communities. This provides for a more balanced assessment of the product and helps ensure that the product will be accepted by local, regional and national regulatory agencies.

- *Fourth party* – Certification by governmental agencies. In some instances, local, regional or national governmental agencies will require that products be evaluated by the agency or a designated representative organization for compliance with regulations for installation, use and operation. Typically, no follow-up monitoring services are provided by the agency. As a result, continued compliance is often left up to the manufacturer.

6.5 Conclusions

In order to ensure an effective overall system that will result in the safe and healthy use of swimming pools and similar recreational environments, it is necessary that these Guidelines inform and be adapted to suit national systems. Figure 6.1 outlines how the Guidelines and the four categories of responsibility outlined within this chapter fit together.

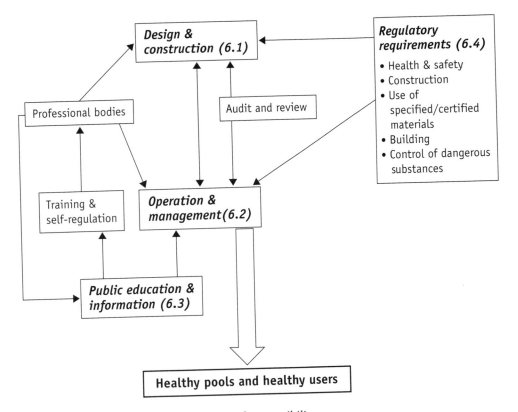

Figure 6.1. Linkages between categories of responsibility

6.6 References

American Red Cross (1995) *Lifeguarding today.* Washington, DC.

Castor Ml, Beach MJ (2004) Reducing illness transmission from disinfected recreational water venues. Swimming, diarrhea and the emergence of a new public health concern. *Pediatric Infectious Disease Journal,* 23(9): 866–870.

Goldhaber GM, de Turck MA (1988) Effectiveness of warning signs: 'familiarity effects'. *Forensic Reports,* 1: 281–301.

Hill V (1984) History of diving accidents. In: *Proceedings of the New South Wales Symposium on Water Safety.* Sydney, New South Wales, Department of Sport and Recreation, pp. 28–33.

ISO (2003) Graphical symbols in safety signs: creating safety signs that everyone comprehends in the same way. *ISO Bulletin,* October: 17–21.

Sport England & Health and Safety Commission (2003) *Managing health and safety in swimming pools,* 3rd ed. Sudbury, Suffolk, UK, HSE Books (HSG Series No. 179).

WHO (2005) *Guide to ship sanitation.* Geneva, World Health Organization, in preparation.

APPENDIX 1
Lifeguards

This appendix relates to people who are trained and positioned at swimming pools to protect water users and who may be paid or voluntary. They may be referred to as lifesavers or lifeguards or given some other title. For simplicity, the term 'lifeguard' has been used throughout this appendix. Box A.1 outlines an example of requirements of a lifeguard, while Box A.2 gives an example of a lifeguard staffing approach.

BOX A.1 EXAMPLES OF REQUIREMENTS OF THE LIFEGUARD AND THEIR DEPLOYMENT

The lifeguard will normally need to be:
- physically fit, have good vision and hearing, be mentally alert and self-disciplined;
- a strong, able and confident swimmer;
- trained and have successfully completed a course of training in the techniques and practices of supervision, rescue and first aid in accordance with a syllabus approved by a recognized training organization.

The deployment of lifeguards would normally take the following into consideration:
- duty spells and structuring of duties — maximum uninterrupted supervision period, working day, programmed breaks;
- lifeguard numbers — dependent on the pool type, size and usage;
- surveillance zones — observation and scanning requirements;
- supervision of changing facilities — showers, toilets, seating and other areas of potential hazard.

Adapted from Sport England & Health and Safety Commission, 2003

Should the pool be used by groups with their own lifeguards, it is important that the criteria that apply to the professional pool lifeguard be equally applied to the groups' lifeguards. Furthermore, there should be documentation on the roles and responsibilities of the groups' lifeguards: the hazards and the potential negative health outcomes associated with those hazards are no less when supervision and management are undertaken by volunteers.

There are a multitude of courses offered for the training and certification of lifeguards. Box A.3 provides examples of some important elements of lifeguard training. Box A.4 provides an example of an international pool lifeguard certificate.

In the United Kingdom, lifeguard numbers may be determined as shown in Table A.1 (Sport England & Health and Safety Commission, 2003).

Table A.1. Lifeguard numbers per square metre of pool

Approximate pool size (m)	Area (m²)	Minimum number of lifeguards (normal)	Minimum number of lifeguards (busy)
20.0 × 8.5	170	1	2
25.0 × 8.5	212	1	2
25.0 × 10.0	250	1	2
25.0 × 12.5	312	2	2
33.3 × 12.5	416	2	3
50.0 × 20.0	1000	4	6

Notes:

1. Where only one lifeguard is on duty, there should be adequate means of summoning assistance rapidly.

2. The 'water area' column can be used as a guide for irregular-shaped pools.

The number of lifeguards required for safety can also be calculated based on sweep time and response time. Some lifeguard training organizations, for example, have created general rules for how quickly they believe a lifeguard should be expected to observe a person in distress within their supervision area and how quickly the lifeguard should be able to reach that person. Based on such rules, training and evaluation, appropriate staffing levels can be derived.

Public interactions
- Responding to inquiries
- Handling suggestions and concerns
- Addressing uncooperative patrons
- Dealing with violence
- Working with diverse cultures
- Accommodating patrons with disabilities

Responsibilities to facility operations
Preventing aquatic injury
Patron surveillance
Facility surveillance
Emergency preparation
Rescue skills
- General procedures
- Entries
- Approaching the victim
- Victims at or near the surface
- Submerged victims
- Multiple victim rescue
- Removal from the water
- Providing emergency care

First aid for injuries
First aid for sudden illnesses
Spinal injury management
- Anatomy and function of the spine
- Recognizing spinal injury
- Caring for spinal injury
- Caring for a victim in deep water
- Spinal injury on land
After an emergency — responsibilities

Adapted from American Red Cross, 1995

BOX A.4 INTERNATIONAL POOL LIFEGUARD CERTIFICATE OF THE INTERNATIONAL LIFE SAVING FEDERATION

For successful recognition for the International Pool Lifeguard Certificate, the candidate must be able to:

LEARNING OUTCOME 1: Perform water-based fitness skills in a pool environment.
Assessment Criteria:
1.1 Swim 50 m in less than 50 s with the head above the water.
1.2 Swim 400 m in less than 8 min without using equipment.
1.3 Retrieve three objects placed 5 m apart in water approximately 2 m deep, or in the deepest end of a pool where the depth is less than 2 m.

LEARNING OUTCOME 2: Demonstrate combined rescue without equipment.
Assessment Criteria:
2.1 Consecutively perform combined rescue technique in the following sequence in less than 2 min:
   - lifesaving entry (stride jump, slide entry); then,
   - 25 m freestyle with head above the water
   - surface dive to adult dummy/person (minimum depth of 1.5 m)
   - lift the dummy/person and tow minimum of 25 m to the edge of pool
   - lift the dummy/person out of the pool.

LEARNING OUTCOME 3: Demonstrate the use of land-based rescue simulation skills.
Assessment Criteria:
3.1 Lift conscious patient and transport them over a minimum distance of 25 m using a recognized patient transport technique.
3.2 Perform simulated rescue using a throwing aid to a conscious victim in the water over a minimum distance of 10 m.

LEARNING OUTCOME 4: Perform emergency response techniques including resuscitation and first-aid techniques.
Assessment Criteria:
4.1 Perform basic patient management techniques, including:
   - diagnosis/check for Dangers, Reaction, Airways, Breathing and Circulation (DRABC)
   - lateral position & patient rollover
   - calling for help
4.2 Perform resuscitation techniques, including:
   - Expired Air Resuscitation (adult, child, infant)

- Cardiopulmonary Resuscitation – CPR (adult, child, infant)
- one- and two-person CPR operation
- set up and apply oxygen equipment

4.3 Identify and perform first-aid techniques for managing injury and emergency, including:
- patient management
- identifying and managing injuries (e.g. shock, fractures, arterial and venal bleeding, spinal injury)

LEARNING OUTCOME 5: Describe medical knowledge about a range of conditions associated with rescues.

Assessment Criteria:

5.1 Describe the application of appropriate emergency treatments in a rescue situation including CPR and spinal management.

5.2 Describe the use of medical equipment in emergency situations.

5.3 Identify regulations pertinent to managing emergency medical situations.

5.4 Identify and list medical services available for support in an emergency medical situation.

LEARNING OUTCOME 6: Choose and plan strategies to manage basic emergencies.

Assessment Criteria:

6.1 Identify and select possible strategies for water rescues and emergencies.

6.2 Identify and solve potential problems for putting plans into place.

6.3 Design a basic emergency management plan.

6.4 Practise emergency management plan.

6.5 Review and modify basic emergency management plan.

LEARNING OUTCOME 7: Identify and describe issues related to the facility/workplace.

Assessment Criteria:

7.1 List the specifications of the pool, including depth, access, use of hot tubs, etc.

7.2 List the nearest available safety services.

7.3 Find and use potential resources for use in rescue.

Assessment Strategy:

These learning outcomes are best assessed using the following common assessment methods:

Observation (personal, video review)

Oral questioning

Written examination (short answer, multiple choice)

Simulated rescue scenario

Range of Variables:

There are a number of variables that will affect the performance and assessment of the learning outcomes. These may include:

Variable	Scope
• Facilities	Swimming pool lengths/depths and measurements (metric/imperial). Use of alternative aquatic locations where pools are not available. Identification of equipment that is available for use.
• Dress	Candidates may be required to wear their recognized uniform.
• Candidates	Candidates will have experience and will be seeking employment or currently employed as a lifeguard.
• Resources	International Life Saving Federation member organizations will list and identify the use of theoretical and practical resources available to them.

Adapted from International Life Saving Federation, 2001

References

American Red Cross (1995) *Lifeguarding today*, Washington, DC.

International Life Saving Federation (2001) *International Pool Lifeguard Certificate*. Approved by ILS Board of Directors, September 2001.

Sport England & Health and Safety Commission (2003) *Managing health and safety in swimming pools*, 3rd ed. Sudbury, Suffolk, UK, HSE Books (HSG Series No. 179).